Who Cares about Health Care?

A Look at the US and Other Nations

Genrich Krasko

ISBN-13:
978-1511718714

To Richard Nixon,
the visionary,
whose 1974 health care reform
was jealously killed by the Left
and too scary for the Right to be resurrected

CONTENTS

Who Cares about Health Care?

ACKNOWLEDGEMENTS

I attribute the conception of this book to an event at Sunday River ski resort in Newry, Maine. On March 9, 2010, I went down a South Ridge slope and was waiting at the lifts for Zeya, my wife, who was coming down. All of a sudden (and I still do not understand what happened) I slipped and fell in horrible pain. In some 30 minutes I was in the nearest hospital– Stephens Memorial – stuffed with morphine. I was lucky to be brought there: this hospital near a popular ski resort had tremendous experience in fixing broken legs and other skiers' bones.

The very next day I had surgery on my left hipbone, which had been corkscrewed by the ski, which had failed to release. The surgery was magic, performed by Dr. Vincent Oliveiro, who made me whole again, collecting my hipbone parts into one with a titanium plate, screws and even a wire.

A week in the hospital followed by another month in a rehab center are where the desire and determination to write a book about health care crystallized. That is why my very first thanks are to Dr. Oliveiro.

My travels through the Internet, learning the history of American health care and attempting to understand how health care systems work in the six countries I had decided to visit, as well as my deep reflection on American health care, took me over three and a half years. And now the book is ready for its readers. For someone who is not a professional writer – and I call myself a layman – writing a book in a language that is not a native one has been a heavy burden.

Therefore, my gratitude goes to the people who made the book readable, stripping it of my "Russian accent" and removing deficiencies in my spelling and grammar. Among them, my deep gratitude goes first to my editor, Judith Cohen, who ceaselessly argued with me, and yet performed the miracle of making the book readable. I am thankful to my friends Woodford McClellan, Edward Besozzi, Theia Vladi, and Dan Varghese who also made corrections in text, as well as Alex Barshevsky and Sergei Sokolovski who helped with graphics. My dear friends Asya Reznikov and Michael Rosenthal used the cartoon by Randy Glasbergen to create a beautiful book cover, and suggested a flashy title.

I am grateful to Dr. Ed Forkos, M.D. for reading a book draft and providing his useful remarks. My deep thanks are to Dr. John Waymouth, a distinguished scientist and thinker, whose encouragement and criticism were of utmost importance to me. I am also grateful to many friends throughout the world who read book drafts and made their suggestions. Among them, I would like to mention correspondence with Regina Naukhovitch of Canada and Ramuald Ripon of France, who helped me better understand the Canadian and French health care systems.

My special thanks are to my dear friend Lev Goldfarb, M.D., for many discussions, constructive criticism, and encouragement.

In spite of my 35-year career as a researcher doing sophisticated computer calculations, I would have been unable to bring this book to its readers without the help of my beloved friends Theia Vladi and Dan Varghese who, as their gift to my 78th birthday, made the book Kindle-readable on Amazon.

Above all, my gratitude to Zeya, my wife, is beyond words.

Genrich L. Krasko
September 2014
Peabody, MA

Introduction

IINTRODUCTION: WHY THIS BOOK?

> Without adequate health care, no one can make full use of his or her talents and opportunities. It is thus just as important that economic, racial and social barriers not stand in the way of good health care as it is to eliminate those barriers to a good education and a good job.
>
> *Richard Nixon*

In 2010, President Obama's Health Care Reform– the Patient Protection and Affordable Care Act (ACA)* – was passed and is now the "Law of the Land." Most people do not know how the new health care system works, though there is an avalanche of sites on the Internet analysing it: GOOGLE alone gives over 2,200,000 links! The idea of the ACA is to provide mandatory national health insurance while leaving intact the foundation of health care – private insurance companies – though partly restricting their grip.

Do we need another book on health care? Now that we will be learning through our own experience how the new health care system works, I thought it would be interesting to compare it with health care systems in other developed countries. That is why I decided to write this book.

This book differs from other books because its source of information is available to everyone: the Internet. The information I have acquired and want to share with my readers is obtainable to anyone who knows how to surf the Web. There are virtually no subjects that cannot be accessed with a few clicks of a mouse.

However, the Internet is an ocean, with its currents and dangerous rocks, and it can sometimes be unreliable. Having found the links they want, people often restrict themselves to what they have read and either accept or reject it. What they find may not be true or objective, or may be outdated (in most cases the

---

* The ACA reform is often called Obamacare. As a derogative label originally used by Republicans it was accepted by Democrats. President Obama even said: "I have no problem with people saying Obama cares." Occasionally, I will be using that label.

link simply does not have the date of its creation, a ridiculous and regretful Internet practice). It is easy to see how Internet users can fall into that trap, especially when they do not have the time or inclination to do more thorough research.

Reading this book will be different from simply surfing the Web because not only have I found interesting and important information, I have selected it critically. I researched sources carefully, sometimes spending hours on a source in order to determine whether the information was not outdated, politically biased, or contradictory.

The book has a great deal of useful information on health care both in America and in six other nations: Canada, France, Germany, Japan, Great Britain, and Israel. I believe that it can be of interest to many. I wanted to show that in other places on earth health care is organized differently. I do not make suggestions of what our health care system should look like. We will go on a journey through different health care systems to explore ideas and practices that inspired other nations. None of the systems we will be visiting is fully appropriate to just copy it here, although careful analysis and a lot of critical thinking will allow us to better understand our own system.

And this book has been written by a layman for laymen. I am a retired Ph. D. physicist (not a physician!). For most of more than 40 years of my career as a scientist I worked in theoretical physics, among the thousands of researchers attempting to understand why metals are strong or brittle, with the goal of developing better, stronger, materials.

The fact that I do not have any education (or, as it would be said today "training") in medical or adjacent fields does make me a layman in this respect. My possible advantage is that I watch the world with an eternal scientist's WHY? And yet, having no expertise in the field I am attempting to venture into, am I eligible to claim your attention?

Freeman Dyson, a renowned theoretical physicist, has written a dozen books outside the area of quantum field theory, in which he is an expert. In one he offers an "apology for a physicist venturing into biology." Over half a century earlier, Erwin Schrödinger, one of the fathers of quantum theory, the foundation of contemporary physics and chemistry, wrote: "Some of us should venture to embark on a synthesis of facts and theories, albeit with second-hand and incomplete knowledge of some of them, and at the risk of making fools of themselves."

I am proud to be in such company. Despite of that risk, I remain optimistic, and I hope my readers will be compassionate.

Introduction

Before we go on our journey, let me discuss the fundamental difference between the health care systems we are going to visit and the one we currently have: in other places, health care is considered as a *right*, whereas in the U.S. it is a *commodity* to be purchased.

Opposing the so-called "individual mandate" – the requirement that health insurance has to be mandatory – conservatives have claimed that as nobody can be forced to purchase anything, no matter what, likewise, purchase of health insurance, as a commodity, cannot be forced on anyone either. The Supreme Court disagreed, and the "individual mandate" of the ACA was upheld.

The left-right dilemma was explicitly formulated in the debate between Barack Obama and John McCain in 2008 as *right* (Obama)[*] vs. *choice* (McCain).

The objection against the first definition has been that as a right, health care is not explicitly mentioned in our Bill of Rights. However, the rights mentioned there are the so-called "enumerated" rights. Apart from the rights explicitly guaranteed in our Constitution, there are other rights, and the Ninth Amendment deals with just this issue.[†] Here is what it says:[1]

> The enumeration in the Constitution of certain rights shall not be construed to deny or disparage others retained by the people.

Among unenumerated rights are the right to privacy, the right to dignity, and many others including Americans' right for K-12 education which is realized by the public school system. No doubt, the right to access health care is among the unenumerated rights that our Constitution does guarantee through the Ninth Amendment. Hence the impressive title of the article: "The 'Silent' Ninth Amendment Gives Americans Rights They Don't Know They Have."[2]

Polarization between Democrats and Republicans has deep ideological roots. In reality, Democrats' *right* presumes the existence of a government-controlled, mandatory health care system, whereas Republicans' *choice* presumes that the decision to purchase or not to purchase health insurance is one's personal matter; therefore the government should have nothing to do with health care, leaving it as a commodity to the market and its forces.

Americans do not want any "socialized" health care because they do not want to pay for anybody's but their own health care. However, as I discuss in the

---

[*] The idea that access to health care is a right was first put forward by Franklin D. Roosevelt in his 1944 State of the Union Address. I mention it in the next chapter.
[†] I discuss the relationship between the First and Ninth Amendments in an essay entitled The Battered First Amendment, The Abandoned Ninth.
(http://www.saynotoboredom.com/the_battered_first_amendment_the_abandoned_ninth.html)

concluding chapter, we did pay, through taxes, for health care and other support systems of 15% Americans – those who are below the Federal Poverty Level (FPL) – even before Obamacare.

Not only do we (the government and states) completely pay for Medicaid – the health care program for low-income and disabled people, we also, through taxes, pay medical expenses for 74% of the services of Medicare, which takes care of our elderly (and does it well!) as well as for emergency rooms and hospital expenses for those who are unable to pay.

In fact this example – supporting the poor and disabled and other humanitarian causes in society – is a good illustration of one of the functions of Social Security. Unfortunately, too often this concept is controversial. How much of social security should a government provide?

How much is too much? "Socialist" Europe has learned that giving too many benefits may become irreversible: people who have become used to them will always be voting against austerity measures and the politicians who support them. In Europe the drastic economic decline is a direct consequence of "too much" social security. In a democratic society there may even exist a point of no return if the people depending on government support are a majority.

As for *health-care-for-all*, as an inalienable part of social security, it is in the consciousness of many Americans, a feature of "socialism." For the very same reason: someone has to pay for actualization of this right for all Americans, and people do not want to be among the "someones." Especially because some pay virtually nothing. Again, the controversial question arises: How much of "free" health care is too much? Is what the ACA mandates too much? We are still too far from achieving health-care-for-all in this country. Americans are strongly polarized with respect to this issue. Would it be good for America or not? A poll shows that 70% of Democrats think that it would be good, whereas 60% of Republicans disagree.[3]

However, not many know that the very first health-care-for-all system as a law was introduced in Germany by Otto von Bismarck[4] over 130 years ago in 1883. Bismarck was a great politician who, within 30 years of being the Prime Minister and then Chancellor of Prussia and then Imperial Chancellor, managed to unite numerous small German fiefdoms and principalities into an empire. He cannot be accused of being a socialist: he was a staunch conservative and a militarist ("War is a natural state of mankind"). However, under his rule some social legislation, unprecedented for their time, were passed, among them the Health Insurance Bill (1883), the Accident Insurance Bill (1884), and the Old Age and Disability Insurance Bill (1889).

The Health Insurance Bill introduced a health care system, which, for many countries, has become a role model for the future. Here are the system's foundations:[5]

- The program provided health care for the majority of German workers.
- The individual local health bureaus were created and managed by a committee elected by the members of each bureau.
- The cost of insurance was divided between employers and employees: 1/3 and 2/3 respectively.
- The minimum payments for medical treatment and sick pay were fixed for up to 13 weeks.

When Bismarck opened debate on the bill in Reichstag, the German parliament in 1881, in his Imperial Message he used the term "practical Christianity." After the bill was passed, Bismarck justified its (and other social legislation's) necessity, writing:

> . . . the actual complaint of the worker is the insecurity of his existence; he is unsure if he will always have work, he is unsure if he will always be healthy and he can predict that he will reach old age and be unable to work. If he falls into poverty, and be that only through prolonged illness, he will find himself totally helpless being on his own, and society currently does not accept any responsibility towards him beyond the usual provisions for the poor, even if he has been working all the time ever so diligently and faithfully.

Though claiming "practical Christianity" as a motivation for his reforms, Bismarck, a pragmatist, also understood that the social stability of a state (to say nothing of an empire) is impossible unless at least a minimal social security has been legislated for the poor. For over 130 years since Bismarck, Germans have never become bankrupt because of their unpaid medical bills.

Bismarck's laws had an important political impact: they were supported by centre-left parties, and cut the ground from under the Social Democrats' feet. After the laws were passed, the latter lost their attraction among workers.[*]

In fact, Bismarck created the first social security on the scale of a state: the provision of a safety net for all.

Bismarck was not the first to introduce social security. In Germany the idea that employment and health care insurance should be linked existed for

---

[*] An unexpected impact: immigration of German workers to America significantly dropped! Workers began migrating to large cities where jobs were more available, and were now "secure" from health care view.

centuries. Medieval professional guilds, which appeared in Europe as early as the 11th or 12th centuries, also provided their members with the support that Bismarck believed was necessary for social stability. Not only did the guilds protect their members from competition with other guilds but they also defended them against town authorities. Guild members cared for the sick and disabled, provided dowries for poor girls, and covered funeral expenses for those who were unable to pay. The funds were collected from all guild members like a tax.[6]

A kind of social security existed as early as in ancient Rome:

> By the second century AD [in Rome] a public medical service was constituted. Public physicians were appointed to various towns and institutions. This practice spread from Italy to Gaul and other provinces. . . . The principal duty of these doctors was to give medical attention to poor citizens. Their salaries were fixed by municipal councillors. They were apparently allowed to accept fees from those who could afford to pay, but they were expected to provide free care for those who could not.[7]

One could call those public services "Ancient Rome–" or "medieval socialism," but they were obviously not. Too often do we forget that compassion, kindness, and concern for others are inalienable qualities of being human. This is the strongest argument in favour of a health-care-for-all system, no matter how it is organized or what it is called.

From the Richard Nixon's quote in one can see that he most probably considered health care as a right, and he was not a liberal. Since Nixon's time the polarization between our two political views has significantly widened. The conservatives moved further to the right, while the liberals moved to the left, thus making any compromise virtually impossible. This polarization created a vacuum in between, a "no-man's land." Unfortunately, this land has been visited too infrequently. And that is where my book belongs. It can be stoned both from the right and the left. I am ready to accept stoning.

The plan of the book is as follows:

Chapter 1: "The History of America's Health Care." Here I share with readers my understanding of how American health care evolved. The struggle between those who wanted a health-care-for-all and those who opposed it was quite dramatic, and a few times the former were close to winning.

In Chapter, 2 I discuss how health-care systems work in six developed democracies: Canada, France, Germany, Japan, Great Britain, and Israel.

Why have I decided to choose these countries?

Introduction

The choice of Canada is obvious: Canada is a whipping boy when it comes to health-care-for-all, and there exists an abundance of lies about its health care system. Besides, Canada's system is a Medicare, "Medicare for all." It is far from ideal, but, in my view, it makes sense to compare their Medicare with ours.

France, according to the World Health Organization (WHO)'s rating of 2000 was No.1 among 190 nations. When this book was already written, in August 2013, Bloomberg issued new rankings of most efficient health care system and the healthiest nations. France was thrown respectively to 19th and 13th places. Yet, The France's health care is an example of non-socialist systems based on a number of non-profit health insurance funds, which cover about 70-80% of costs, leaving room for for-profit supplemental insurers.

Visiting Germany is interesting because for more than a century Germany has had a health care system grounded in Otto von Bismarck's 1883 revolutionary universal health care reform, which Bismarck characterized as "practical Christianity." It was the very first system to have the health care cost split between employees (two-thirds) and employers (one–third). From the very beginning it covered the great majority of German workers.

Japan is fascinating because, like the legendary phoenix bird, it was born anew after the WWII devastation, and created a flourishing economy and a role-model democracy. Its health care system is a Bismarckian one, with additional and original features of its own.

Great Britain has a health care system that could be called socialized. The majority of doctors are government employees either directly, such as hospital doctors, or through subcontracting, like primary care physicians.

And finally, there is Israel. In spite of an extremely difficult social and political situation, this country has developed its own specific health care system on par with the best.

In Chapter 3, I briefly review President Obama's health care reform, still shrouded in fog, and I attempt to be as objective as possible. The chapter answers some "foggy" questions, which are only gradually beginning to surface today.

The next chapter, "Where Are We? America's Health Care Today," is a reflection on the current American health care situation as thinking and curious individual sees it. With the persistence of a former scientist, I analyze our health care expenses. I introduce an *Affluence Factor*: the ratio of GDP of America to the GDPs of other nations. This allows me to compare "apples to apples," America's health care expenses with those of other nations, if the other nations were as affluent as we are. I also discuss the most significant failures of our health care system: "head maladies" (vision, dentistry, and psychiatry), maternity services, and long-term health care. Detailed discussion of two government programs, Medicaid and Medicare, may be of interest to many. Too often the non–poor and non–elderly do not understand how these programs work. What I have discovered discussing America's health care today may be an eye-opener to some readers.

In the concluding chapter, "How Are We Different?" a detailed table of health-care indicators is compiled in order to summarize how the American health care system differs from those of the aforementioned six countries, even though in other chapters, where appropriate, I have already compared the health care systems. In particular, discussing health care economics, the application of the *Affluence Factors,* introduced in the previous chapter, shows that the widely held belief that America greatly overspends on health care compared to other nations is not entirely correct, although some 30% of our expenses could have been avoided. I also discuss what an alternative to Obamacare reform might have been.

Finally, in the Appendix I share with my readers a document that I unexpectedly found forgotten under the layers of decades of political struggle in America: Richard Nixon's "Special Message to the Congress" of February 6, 1974,[8] proposing a comprehensive health insurance plan which, almost 40 years ago, might have solved our health care problems, but was killed; neither the Republicans nor the Democrats cared to resurrect it.

I have a request: Before reading the book, please return to the epigraph to this Introduction: an excerpt from Richard Nixon's Message to Congress. Give yourself a few moments to read and think about what he said, and compare it with what you hear too often these days.

1. HISTORY OF HEALTH CARE IN AMERIKA

> I like the dreams of the future better
> than the history of the past.
> *Thomas Jefferson*

Health care in America as a culture of insurance policies has its own history. Of course, it did not always exist. New immigrants leaving ships at Ellis Island could rely only on themselves if they got sick. They called a doctor or were taken to a hospital and they paid from their own pockets.

The need for insurance in case of injury or sickness was perceived relatively early in our history. During the Civil War, individual health insurance could be purchased that would cover injuries sustained while traveling by steamboat or train as these new means of transportations were believed to be unsafe. The earliest group insurance policies that covered accidents originated in 1887 in Massachusetts. By the beginning of the twentieth century, disability insurance that covered a wide range of injuries and illnesses had evolved.

Before 1920, medicine was rather primitive: most diseases were poorly understood. The means of diagnosis were few and restricted: although X-ray examinations were used, but they were dangerous to both patients and doctors because of radiation dosages much higher than those used today; blood-pressure measuring devices existed; and blood tests were available, although they were not as sophisticated as they are at present. And yet, the doctor's main tool was a stethoscope.

Doctors attended patients primarily in their homes and treated them there. Even surgeries were often performed in homes. Antiseptics were not yet fully developed and hospitals were nothing like those we know today. In the nineteenth and the first quarter of the twentieth century, health care was not a "major industry," and played no significant role in the American market.

Before 1904, medical education in America was mostly unregulated. In 1904 the Council for Medical Education, created by the American Medical Association (AMA), introduced standards for licensing new doctors. Before 1910, 90% of doctors either had no college education or had attended substandard medical schools, and had no license to practice medicine. In 1910, the Fletcher Report (commissioned by the AMA and the Carnegie Foundation) was published,[1] which suggested that a high school diploma and at least two years of college should be required before admittance to a medical school, and that medical school education should last four years. Most of Fletcher's recommendations were accepted by the AMA and medical schools in the U.S.

In a sense, Fletcher's report was a revolution. It claimed that there were too many unqualified medical schools, and too few qualified doctors. In the following years, due to the increased requirements for doctors' training, the number of medical schools (mostly affiliated with universities) significantly shrank. For this reason, though the number of MDs decreased by almost half, their quality increased to match the higher standards. In 1913 the American College of Surgeons was founded which imposed stringent accreditation standards for hospitals. In 1918, only 13% of large hospitals were accredited by the ACS; by 1932, 93% of hospitals became accredited.

The higher standards of medical education resulted in increasing its cost, thus making it accessible only to the privileged. The cost of health care begins to climb.

Before the "Fletcher revolution," doctors did not charge patients high fees, knowing that their art was not perfect, and that the care they provided was often primitive. Typically, physicians did not earn a lot: in 1913 their annual income was $500 to $700, which was not much higher than that of manual laborers. America then was not as rich as it is today. The middle class was in its infancy. Most people were poor, and could not pay much even if doctors were to demand higher fees. Thus health care was not expensive.

Due to the primitive state of medical technology before 1920, most people spent very little on medical needs. In fact, the chief problem with an illness was not the expense of medical care, but rather the fact that sick people didn't get paid because they couldn't work. In the State of Illinois in 1919, lost wages due to illnesses were four times larger than the cost of treating those illnesses.[2] Health insurance was therefore not a necessity for most people. Rather, they preferred to purchase "sickness" insurance – like today's disability insurance – to guarantee some income in case of illness.

The third decade of the twentieth century brought revolutionary changes. It was the beginning of the gradual substitution of medical science for the "art" of the physician. New medical procedures and drugs were developed and a network of hospitals evolved, including specialty hospitals and treatment centers like Children's Hospital in Boston, Cancer Hospital in New York City, and Chinese Hospital in San Francisco.

As happens in revolutions, these radical changes were the accumulation of previous achievements. The time has come for them to go to the forefront.

Here are the milestones in medical science and technology that made possible the break-throughs in American medicine that occurred by the first half of the twentieth century.[2]

1850 - 1870: Louis Pasteur, Joseph Lister and others develop an understanding of bacteriology, antisepsis, and immunology.

1870 - 1910: Various infectious agents are identified, including those causing syphilis, typhus, pneumococcus, and malaria. The diphtheria antitoxin is developed.

1887: S.S.K. von Basch invents the instrument for measuring blood pressure.

1895: Wilhelm Roentgen discovers x-rays.

1903: Willem Einthoven develops the first electrocardiograph.

1910: Salvarsan becomes the first drug for the treatment of syphilis that wipes out the disease without injuring the patient.

1917: Cholera and typhus vaccine developed

1920s: Insulin is isolated as a pancreatic extract.

1923: Diphtheria vaccine is developed.

1926: Pertussis vaccine is developed.
1927: Tuberculosis (BCG) and tetanus vaccine is developed.
1928: Alexander Fleming discovers penicillin (Nobel Prize). (Large-scale production of synthetic penicillin begins in 1946.)

1930s: Sulphonamides are discovered and are used successfully in treating bacterial diseases.

1928: Adolf Windhous discovers vitamin D (Nobel Prize).

1928: The first ventilator (the iron lung) is used in Boston's Children's Hospital.

1930: Karl Landsteiner identifies human blood types (Nobel Prize).

Can we imagine today's first-aid kit without Band-Aids? They were invented by a nurse in 1921.

In 1918 the United States stood 17th out of 20 nations in mortality rates. In the 1920s American life expectancy began to climb.

Who Cares about Health Care?

Because of the development of new techniques that most doctors' offices could not afford or didn't know how to use, hospitals began to spread throughout the country. Also, because of the growth of industry accompanied by increased urbanization, people lived in smaller homes or apartments. This made treating acute illnesses at home impossible. The proliferation of hospitals equipped with more advanced means of treating illnesses encouraged people to abandon home treatment. In the 1920s, patients, apart from hoping to be cured, began feeling that medicine was changing significantly, becoming different: more precise, more scientific, and thus more effective. The cost of health care began to climb.

The estimates done in 1925 claimed that at least 2% of entire population was constantly sick, and there was an average seven days loss of wages per person. The average cost of medical care (the services of doctors, nurses, hospitals, and medicines) was estimated to be about $10 per capita, and the loss of wages due to illness was $12, making the total expenditure $22. That was a good deal of money. The cost of care was almost equal to the loss of wages, while, as I mentioned, in 1919 medical expenditures were only one fourth of the lost wages due to illness.

Among the causes of the increased costs these were the most significant:

• Shifting medical care from homes to hospitals with advanced technology: In 1929, an American family's medical bills were about $108, 14% of which were for hospital stays. For an urban family making $2,000 to $3,000 per year the medical bill was only $67 if there was no hospitalization; otherwise it jumped to $261. Hospital costs were rising, reaching close to 40% of a family's expenses by 1934.[2]

• Increased qualification of physicians: As mentioned above, following the requests from the AMA's Council of Medical Education, the requirements for medical licensure were raised and standardized. With some schools unable to meet the new standards, the number of medical schools in the United States dropped from 131 in 1910 to 95 in 1915. By 1922, the number had fallen even further to 81. The decreased supply resulted in increased demand, increased competition among physicians, and thus higher costs for their services.

• The cost of transportation of the sick to the place of service (a doctor's office or a hospital) – even by public transport in cities, but by much more expensive automobile in rural areas – could significantly contribute to the cost of health care.

These increased medical costs spurred the development of health insurance.

As I mentioned in the Introduction, the concept of health insurance originated in Europe in medieval times as a form of professional guild insurance. Modern health insurance began in Germany with von Bismarck's reforms of 1983. By 1912 most European nations already had health insurances similar to Bismarck's concepts.

In America, in the late nineteenth and early twentieth centuries, a kind of health insurance was available. There were six types of insurance:

– fraternal societies and mutual benefit associations
– contract physicians*
– private physician plans
– county medical bureau† plans
– hospital service plans, and
– group insurance plans operated by private commercial insurance companies.

Thus, by the late 1920s when the "medical revolution" began, America did have a health insurance industry, although it did not yet play a significant role in the economy.

However, before the period in question, private companies were reluctant to go into the health insurance business. Capitalism, which was developing by gigantic steps conquering America, and making the laws of the market the most prominent laws of the land, was also a major factor in preventing development of a comprehensive health insurance system. Those private companies did not believe that health was an insurable commodity because, unlike a house that has burned down where no proof of destruction is needed, coverage of a "sick" person does not allow for the reliable calculation of risks and corresponding premiums. The "lyrics of this song" (still sung today) were expressed in 1919 by *The Insurance Monitor*: "The opportunities for fraud [in health insurance] upset all statistical calculations. . . . Health and sickness are vague terms open to endless construction. Death is clearly defined, but to say what shall constitute such loss of health as will justify insurance compensation is no easy task."[2]

There is no mention here of "practical Christianity," the central moral argument of Bismarck's 1883 reform. Now I will tell the story of the political

---

* From 1908 – 1912 the first "contract doctor" system, organized by Dr. Raymond G. Taylor, was operational and took care of 10,000 workers at the Los Angeles Aqueduct project.
† First organized in 1917, medical bureaus were groups of physicians who, for a monthly fee, provided medical care to employees of specific businesses. They were the precursers of Blue Shield. (I appreciate the personal correspondence with Professors J. Erien and R. LaPorte of the University of Pittsburgh.)

wars involving health insurance that were waged during the following decades and up to our time.

In the beginning of the twentieth century, in spite of the variety of insurance options available, a large percentage of Americans did not have health insurance, mostly because they actually needed loss of income, rather than health insurance. As a result, their access to quality medical care was limited.

I have already mentioned that an average physician at that time could hardly make a living. That was the second factor that created a push for a kind of mandatory health insurance.

The beginning of the twentieth century is known as the Progressive Era, which saw reformers' activity directed at improving workers'social conditions. President Theodore Roosevelt (1901-1909) was a "progressive" president. He believed that the country could be strong only if people were healthy and not poor. Therefore he supported social insurance, including health insurance. National health insurance was on his agenda. However, in 1912 he was defeated by Woodrow Wilson, and in the following years the main push for reform was not made by the government.

The most influential political force and the most powerful advocate of reform was an organization called the Progressive Movement in American Policies. From 1915 to1920, this organization was instrumental in achieving major improvements in regulating child labor, quality of food and drugs, minimum wages, and conditions in the workplace. Creating some type of government-supported mandatory health insurance was a natural outgrowth of the organization's activities. However, the major push for reform came from the American Association of Labor Legislation (AALL), a private organization that had been instrumental in fighting unacceptable health conditions in the workplace in a number of industries.

AALL sent a commission to Europe to study firsthand the state-supported health plans in Germany and England. As early as 1915, the AALL suggested a health insurance plan that would cover the vast majority of American workers.[3] The cost for this package broke down as follows: 40% contributed each by the employer and the employee, with the balance of 20% paid by the government. In 1917, the American medical community's first response to the AALL plan was positive.

The AMA – the voice of American doctors – supported it. (It reversed its position in 1920.) Next was an attempt to pass legislation. The first "guinea pigs" were the states of New York, Massachusetts, and New Jersey.

In New York, the bill originally met with resistance by physicians because it rejected the fee for service principle and the right of the patient to choose a physician. Eventually, after compromises, the bill was endorsed by a few medical organizations but was never passed.

Unexpectedly, a leader of the American Federation of Labor, Samuel Gompers, stated before the U.S House of Representatives that "the workers would rather take care of themselves than rely on the assistance of the federal government." However, as could have been expected, stronger opposition to a federally funded health care system came from a group of private insurance companies who fought tooth and nail to defend their lucrative business, which would evaporate should the government become actively involved in health care. In order to block the passage of any health care legislation, these companies pooled their resources and created the Insurance Economic Society of America (IESA), which became instrumental in financing and lobbying organizations opposing the health care legislation.

Any progress towards developing a meaningful health care system in America was blocked by the confrontation between the AALL and the IESA. However, in 1917, when America entered World War I, the confrontation became irrelevant. Because of strong anti-German sentiment, even the idea of copying anything German was deemed unpatriotic.The Germans' mandatory health-care-for-all concept was believed to be un-American and thus had to be prohibited.

In 1917, the American medical establishment vehemently opposed health insurance legislation. The medical societies – the AMA foremost among them – believed that they would be able to kill any legislation of federally funded insurance. Using strong anti-German sentiments, medical societies throughout America launched a propaganda campaign warning the public about the "evil" of state health insurance. "Even the federal government, through the propaganda activities of the Creel Committee on Public Information, claimed that the concept of state health insurance was a German doctrine that was a 'fraud' against American workers."

After the war, America was engulfed in the "Red Scare." The Russian Communist Revolution, the wide-scale labor strikes, and civil rights unrest in 1919-1920 made advancement of any ideas even slightly smelling of socialism impossible. In 1920 the AMA became openly hostile to a mandatory government-supported system. President Warren G. Harding was elected in 1920, running on a strong anti-insurance platform. The new era had begun.

The main factors that caused the defeat of the reformers were as follows.

The animosity towards Germany played a major role. The second factor was the unwillingness of physicians to accept any mandatory health insurance that would negatively affect their incomes. The social atmosphere after the war had changed: the pre-war progressive era of liberal thinking was over. Unlike in Europe, there was no support of socialist ideas in health care among the low-income population (which needed reliable health insurance more than any others). Added to that was the aggressive lobbying and anti-reform propaganda of the medical organizations and private insurance companies.

This nearly ten-year-long period culminated in the Great Depression of 1929, which brought Franklin Delano Roosevelt to the presidency and the New Deal. However, the important events in American health care happened even before FDR's first hundred days.

What I mean is the emergence of two programs, still the backbone of the health insurance industry in our time: Blue Cross and Blue Shield. These programs were created as voluntary insurance agencies that could meet doctors' and hospitals' economic needs while at the same time prevent government intervention. Both were originated by a medical profession that was forced to change its attitude towards health insurance. And for that there were serious reasons.

With the Depression, America's economy collapsed. With it tumbled the economic security of the medical profession. In 1929-1930, in the South, the average income of an internist fell by nearly 50%. Between 1929 and 1930, average hospital receipts plummeted from more than $200 per patient to less than $60.[4] The hospital occupancy rate also declined: in private hospitals, on average, only 62% of beds were occupied.

By 1929, a new idea of how to save hospitals crystalized. The Baylor Univesrsity Hospital in Waco, Texas, agreed to enroll patients (1250 Dallas public school teachers) in an inexpensive prepaid plan. Such a system was advantageous for both hospitals and patients: it did not interfere with patients' rights to choose their own doctors and hospitals. Soon other hospitals followed suit. In 1932 a number of hospitals in Sacramento, California, created a multi-hospital prepaid insurance plan. Such plans rapidly spread across America.

Officially, the Blue Cross plan was born and adopted by the American Hospital Association (AHA) in 1933. By 1938, the AHA established a policy for national Blue Cross. Each group of local hospitals could set its own fee schedule so that there would be no competition among local Blue Cross hospitals.

Because there were no commercial companies behind Blue Cross plans, they were allowed to act as non-profit organizations with tax-exempt status and did not need to comply with complicated regulations for insurance companies. For that, however, they had to pay by being overseen by state governments.

The emergence of Blue Cross was, unwittingly, a menace to private physicians. Their voice, the AMA, had two objectives: to protect doctors from competition with Blue Cross and to provide an alternative to mandatory insurance. In 1934 the AMA formulated ten principles that became the foundation of a new insurance plan. An important provision was that voluntary health insurance would remain under the control of physicians, rather than a non-medical bureaucracy. The physicians also wanted to be able to bill patients discriminately, that is, charge different rates to different patients based on their ability to pay. This plan was called Blue Shield.

Like Blue Cross, the new plans were tax exempt and were relieved from the bureaucratic hassles that the insurance companies had to deal with. The first such prepayment plan was offered in California in 1939 under the name the California Physicians' Services. It was opened for people earning less than $3,000/year and provided physicians' services for $1.70 per month per person. The AMA encouraged creating prepayment plans through state and local medical societies. Ultimately, by 1946, all such plans joined to form the giant Blue Shield that we have today. The two Blue plans differed significantly. One of Blue Cross's primary goals was to provide health care through hospitals for the entire community; Blue Shield's objective was mainly to guarantee physicians adequate income while controlling health care delivery and preventing the government from interfering.

Here I should also mention the creation, at the height of the Great Depression, a first "pre-payment" system. An inspired doctor, Sidney Garfield, organized the treatment of sick and injured people working for the Colorado River Aqueduct Project. The original system was simple: for 5 cents a day, workers had basic coverage. For another 5 cents a day non–job-related medical problems were covered. Thousands of people enrolled. With the beginning of WWII the system was expanded by industrialist Henry J. Kaiser, with the hub at Kaiser Shipyards in Richmond, California. The "Kaiser Permanente" system officially opened in 1945, and became very popular in California, with the enrollment of hundreds of thousands of people. Today it is a partnership of non-profit Kaiser Foundation Health Plan and Hospitals and the Permanente Medical Groups.[5]

The development of the American health care system that I am going to discuss now is the legacy of thirteen American presidents. A concise review of this development as seen through their State of the Union Addresses, can be found in the site *State of the Union and Health Care: 100 Years of Good Intentions*.[6]

With the election of Franklin D. Roosevelt as the 32nd president in 1933, an era of social legislation began. His twelve-year tenure all but changed America for at least four decades, if not for good. He led America through the end of the

Great Depression and World War II, and spurred a number of important social policies, including the series of economic programs known as the New Deal.[7]

The New Deal was a response to the Great Depression and focused on "three r's:" relief, recovery and reform. Government-controlled health care reform was also on the agenda. FDR hoped that health legislation could pass within an overall social legislation package.

One might have thought that after the Great Depression the conditions for passing a health-care-for-all legislation were ideal. However, with millions without jobs, unemployment insurance and old age benefits had higher priority. Therefore the health insurance provision was not included in the 1935 Social Security Bill. The AMA was against the bill; including health care might have killed it altogether.

There was one more attempt to pass health care legislation.

The New Deal social reform forces renewed their efforts to promote mandatory health insurance in 1938 by sponsoring the National Health Conference in Washington, D.C., thus focusing national attention on the need for compulsory health insurance to assure access to medical care for a large segment of the American public. To meet this new challenge, the AMA and the private insurance companies increased their lobbying efforts in Congress and their attacks nationally through the newspapers, warning the public about the supposed evil of mandatory government-funded health insurance.

Their efforts were successful. In 1939 the last attempt of New Dealers to pass federally funded health insurance legislation (the Wagner Health Bill) was soundly defeated in Congress. Then WWII began, and health insurance reform was pushed to the back burner.

However, in 1943, despite the war, another attempt was made – the Wagner-Murray-Dingell Bill. This bill's intent was that the health care system would be financed through payroll deductions rather than taxes and federal grants. Though there was wide national debate, the bill was never passed, although it was introduced in every congressional session for the next 14 years!

In his 1944 State of the Union Address FDR proposed *The Second Bill of Rights* as a necessary extension of the First Bill of Rights, the foundation of the American Constitution. FDR claimed that all people have "the right to adequate medical care and the opportunity to achieve and enjoy good health."[8] He was the first president to explicitly insist that medical care is a right, without which "pursuit of happiness" is impossible.

After FDR died, Harry Truman became president (1945-1953). By 1945 World War II was over and the Cold War dawned. America began its new economic growth, and the health care issue grew into a problem of national importance. Truman insisted that America needs a "national system of payment for medical care based on well-tried insurance principles. . . . Our ultimate aim must be a comprehensive insurance system to protect all our people equally against insecurity and ill health."[9] He wholeheartedly supported national health insurance in spite of the strong anti-Communist mood in the country. In the atmosphere of the Cold War, the opposition to reform used socialized medicine as a symbolic issue in the growing crusade against Communist influence in America. The story of Truman's attempt to accomplish the reform is quite dramatic.

In 1945, Truman was strongly committed to a universal comprehensive health insurance plan. It differed from FDR's 1938 program, which had proposed separate medical care for the poor. Truman's plan included everyone equally but was not to be interpreted as socialized medicine. He abandoned the funeral benefit, which had helped defeat national insurance in the Progressive Era. The reaction of Congress was mixed. The chairman of the House Committee, an anti-union conservative, refused to hold hearings. Senior Republican Senator Robert A. Taft declared, "I consider it socialism. It is to my mind the most socialistic measure this Congress has ever had before it." Taft's reaction was extreme. He said that compulsory health insurance came right out of the Soviet constitution and walked out of the hearings. The AMA, the American Hospital Association, the American Bar Association, and most of the nation's press hated the plan unequivocally. The AMA claimed it would make doctors slaves, even though Truman emphasized that doctors would be able to choose their method of payment.

The Republican-controlled Congress of 1946 wanted no part of national health insurance, believing that it was part of a large socialist scheme. In response, Truman advocated a national health bill with even more passion in the 1948 election. After his surprise victory in 1948, the AMA was mobilized. They expressed their opposition to national health insurance by assessing each of their members an extra $25. In 1945 they spent $1.5 million on lobbying efforts. One of their pamphlets said, "Would socialized medicine lead to socialization of other phases of life? Lenin thought so." He declared that socialized medicine is the keystone to the arch of the socialist state. The AMA and its supporters were successful in linking socialism with national health insurance and thus Truman's plan died in a congressional committee. Along with growing anti-Communist feeling in the late 1940s and the start of the Korean War national health insurance became vanishingly improbable.

Meanwhile, in the 1940s and '50s, commercial insurance companies began aggressively entering the health care market. What had before scared the insurance companies from entering the market was so-called adverse selection, or, more simply, cheating by the sick that would prevent the business from being profitable. Now they were encouraged by the success of Blue Cross and Blue Shield.

The adverse selection problem could be easily overcome if health insurance were provided to groups of employees only: then relatively young, healthy people in groups would be insured. Commercial health insurance companies then began aggressively moving into the health insurance market, which boomed. In the 1940s total enrollment was only 20,662,000; it exploded to nearly 142,334,000 in 1950.[2]

By the 1950s, commercial or Blue Cross–Blue Shield group insurance through employers became widespread and popular. Through Congress and the Supreme Court, government encouraged group health insurance. Beginning with the 1943 administrative ruling and eventually codified in 1954 by the IRS, employers' contributions to employees' health plans were not taxed and these contributions were also exempt from employees' taxable income.

President Dwight D. Eisenhower's two terms as President (1953-1961) were relatively quiet (if one disregards the raging Cold War and the infamous Senator McCarthy's witch-hunt). However, beginning in 1952, hospitals' and physicians' bills begin escalating and have not stopped escalating since. One of the factors was definitely the further advances in medical technology, making treatments more expensive. Was it also because for-profit companies entered the market?

In 1956, addressing Congress, Eisenhower said: "We must aid in cushioning the heavy and rising costs of illness and hospitalization to individuals and families . . . Plans should be evolved to improve protection against the costs of prolonged or severe illness. These measures will help reduce the dollar barrier between many Americans and the benefits of modern medical care."[10] Under public pressure, and in order to prevent a more radical health care reform, the AMA joined Eisenhower administration in compiling legislation that would relieve, though only partially, the health care system's economic pressure. The Kerr-Mills bill was passed in 1960. It gave the states federal funding to cover the health care cost of the growing elderly population. The AMA could not tolerate anything more radical and in 1961 it was instrumental in killing the King-Anderson Bill, which would have allowed payments for elderly hospitalization through the social security system.

The short and tragic Kennedy presidency (1961-1963), in spite of his New Frontier programs, was unable to achieve any breakthrough in passing federally funded health care insurance. All his bills were defeated in Congress. It was Lyndon B. Johnson (1963-1969), JFK's successor, who was able to achieve what Roosevelt, Truman, and Kennedy had failed to achieve.

In 1964, Johnson's first effort, the hospitalization plan, was defeated in Congress. However, that very year his sweeping victory as an elected president brought an extremely liberal Democratic majority to the House and Senate, dramatically changing the political scene. Democrats controlled the House by 2:1, and had 32 more seats in the Senate than Republicans.

For decades, the opposition to any form of nationalized health care was like a brick wall. However, the creation of Medicaid and Medicare was a significant breakthrough. Here is how the situation looked before that breakthrough.

 By 1958, nearly 75% of Americans had some form of private health insurance coverage. The medical profession had prevented government's intervention by helping to implement a successful system of voluntary health insurance plans. The AMA opposed any nationalized health insurance programs, calling such proposals socialistic and bound to interfere with physician income and the doctor-patient relationship. It had played a crucial role in defeating proposals for nationalized health insurance in 1935 and later, in 1949, in defeating the proposed Murray-Wagner-Dingell (MWD) bill. Like a union, the AMA charged every physician who was a member $25 for their lobbying efforts.[2]

At that time $25 was no small amount. Senator Barry Goldwater wrote in 1964: "Having given our pensioners their medical care in kind, why not food baskets, why not public housing accommodations, why not vacation resorts, why not a ration of cigarettes for those who smoke and of beer for those who drink?"[11]

However, no matter how much health care for all was hated, a new era, the era of the Great Society, had begun[12] and would further expand under the presidencies of Richard Nixon and Gerald Ford.

To the proponents of universal health insurance, the idea to focus first on those over the age of 65 was a smart strategy. Now its opponents could no longer insist that the elderly are affluent enough to pay for old-age health care. Now the old maxim "If you can't beat them, join them!" seemed appropriate. Therefore the opponents switched their focus from opposing the bill to creating new forms of it: Republican committee member John Byrnes' version, the AMA version, and Medicare, the adminstration's version. According to Byrnes, doctors' services and medications should be paid for by the government and the aged could receive coverage on a voluntary basis. Elderly patients in need would receive financing from the government, which would be scaled to the amount of their Social Security cash benefits. Eldercare, an AMA proposal, would cover physicians' charges, surgery, medications, nursing home costs, x-rays and lab services and would also be paid for by the government. Byrnes' bill, Eldercare, and Medicare were all presented to the Ways and Means Committee.

Who Cares about Health Care?

In the 1965 deliberations, all AMA proposals were rejected. Ways and Means chair Wilbur Mills and his committee drafted the bill that became law, combining Byrnes' concepts and Medicare. Part of Byrnes' proposal included lowering taxes. This had to be amended because the program's estimated costs necessitated higher taxes.

The first ever government health program – Medicare – was passed in Congress as part of the Social Security Act[13] and was signed by Lyndon B. Johnson into law on July 30, 1965 in Independence, Missouri, the home-town of former president Truman. At the bill signing ceremony, Truman and his wife Bess were handed Medicare cards numbers one and two. Johnson credited Truman with "planting the seeds of compassion and duty which have today flowered into care for the sick and serenity for the fearful."

Medicare was a federal program and consisted of parts A and B. Part A was a mandatory hospital insurance program in which the elderly would have to be automatically enrolled after the age of 65. It was to be financed through payroll deduction, and in this sense was "free." Part B would cover physicians' services. Part B was not free: the necessary funds would have to be collected from the recipients' monthly payments, income taxes and interest from the Medicare Trust Fund. As one can see, today's Medicare's foundations have not changed.*

Unexpectedly for physicians, having agreed to accept Medicare patients, they actually benefited significantly. The legislation established that physicians were to be reimbursed according to "usual, customary, and reasonable rates," which was not bad. Also, patients could be directly billed by physicians, with Medicare later reimbursing them. Physicians could also bill discriminately (on which they also insisted), charging or not charging patients in excess of Medicare payments according to their bills. (This was later prohibited.) As a result, physicians' incomes grew significantly. Hospitals also greatly benefited; they did not have to pay for charity patients: the government reimbursed these expenses. In 1966 Medicare enrolled 19.1 million people; by 1999 the enrollment grew to 39.5 million.

Another program, Medicaid, was also a part of the 1965 Social Security Act.[14] This program was to cover all aspects of health care (hospitals, physicians, testing, etc.) for definite categories of low income or disabled people.

Medicaid was to be jointly funded by the federal government and states. Participation of states in the program was voluntary. Arizona was the last to join in 1988. Medicaid is a means-treated program: in order to be eligible, a

---

* I discuss Medicaid and Medicare in detail in Chapter 4.

person or a family must prove that their income is within certain limits and must satisfy definite criteria. Among those covered were low-income children without parental support, their care-giver relatives, the blind, and people with disabilities. The eligibility criteria varied from state to state.

These are the key milestones in Medicare and Medicaid history from the years 1965 through 1972:

•1965--Medicare and Medicaid were enacted as Title XVIII and Title XIX of the Social Security Act, extending health coverage to almost all Americans age 65 or over (e.g., those receiving retirement benefits from Social Security or the Railroad Retirement Board), and providing health care services to low income people, and also to low-income children deprived of parental support, their caretaker relatives, the elderly, the blind, and individuals with disabilities.

•1966—Medicare was implemented on July 1, serving more than 19 million individuals. Medicaid funding was available to states starting January 1, 1966; the program was phased in by states over a several-year period.

•1967—An Early and Periodic Screening, Diagnosis, and Treatment (EPSDT) comprehensive health services benefit for all Medicaid children under age 21 was established.

•1972—Medicare eligibility was extended to 2 million individuals under age 65 with long-term disabilities and to individuals with end-stage renal disease (ESRD). Medicare was given the authority to conduct demonstration programs.[15]

Medicaid eligibility for elderly, blind, and disabled residents of a state could be linked to eligibility for the newly enacted Federal Supplemental Security Income Program (SSI). Eighteen million individuals were covered by Medicaid when the program was implemented.

In 1969 Richard Nixon became the 37th president. Congress belonged to the Democrats, with whom Nixon's relations were strained. For a long time, Nixon has been a whipping boy in America. Unfortunately, Watergate has overshadowed his achievements, which were many. One achievement is worth mentioning in this context.

Would anybody today (especially the young) believe that a Republican president could have suggested a "socialist" health care reform? But Nixon, a staunch conservative, did. In February of 1974, in the middle of Watergate, Nixon sent a message to Congress suggesting aComprehensive Health

Insurance Plan (CHIP*). Here it is in Nixon's own words:

> Three years ago, I proposed a major health insurance program to the Congress, seeking to guarantee adequate financing of health care on a nationwide basis. That proposal generated widespread discussion and useful debate. But no legislation reached my desk.
>
> Early last year, I directed the Secretary of Health, Education, and Welfare to prepare a new and improved plan for comprehensive health insurance. That plan, as I indicated in my State of the Union message, has been developed and I am presenting it to the Congress today. I urge its enactment as soon as possible.
>
> The plan is organized around seven principles:
>
> First, it offers every American an opportunity to obtain a balanced, comprehensive range of health insurance benefits;
>
> Second, it will cost no American more than he can afford to pay;
>
> Third, it builds on the strength and diversity of our existing public and private systems of health financing and harmonizes them into an overall system;
>
> Fourth, it uses public funds only where needed and requires no new Federal taxes;
>
> Fifth, it would maintain freedom of choice by patients and ensure that doctors work for their patient, not for the Federal Government.
>
> Sixth, it encourages more effective use of our health care resources;
>
> And finally, it is organized so that all parties would have a direct stake in making the system work--consumer, provider, insurer, State governments and the Federal Government. [16]

If one wants to understand not just the history of health care reforms, but today's situation as well, one should read the full document: just 8 pages. It can be found in this book's Appendix.

What happened to that proposal? Of course it was killed. Ben Stein, a writer, lawyer and commentator, as well as a former speechwriter for Nixon and Ford, wrote recently:

---

* Not to be confused with another CHIP – Children's Healt Insurance Program – created in 1997 under the Clinton administration

In many ways, the bill was far more "socialist" than what Mr. Obama has proposed. It certainly involved a far larger swath of state and federal government power over health care. Please remember that this was 36 years ago, when middle-class Americans still had some slight faith that government was on their side.

My point is not whether or not Mr. Nixon's plan was better than Mr. Obama's. In fact, they have many points in common.

My only point is that if you want to call someone a visionary, if you want to call someone compassionate, if you want to note that someone was a foe of inequality and a friend to mercy, think of Richard Nixon, with a host of problems of his own the likes of which Mr. Obama cannot imagine, reaching out to the poor and the uninsured to help.

The plan, of course, was killed dead by the Democrats, led by Edward Kennedy, who later regretted what he had done. Still, attention must be paid to a prophet without honor in his own land.[17]

The prophet has been stoned. If not for his fatal Watergate misstep, he probably would have re-submitted CHIP and quite possibly, it would have passed. Then for the past 30 years, America would have had a comprehensive health care system and would not need new "prophets."

Unfortunately, the continuation of the health care story is no less scandalous. In 1977 Jimmy Carter became President. Four months later he sent to Congress his Health Care Legislation Message. It consisted of two parts: the Hospital Cost Containment Act and the Child Health Assessment Program (CHAP).

Commenting on the first program, the Message says: [18]

This legislation is not a wage-price control program. It places no restrictions on the hospital's ability to determine its charges for any particular service. It places no limit on the size of any wage demand or settlement. The program establishes an overall limit on the rate of increase in reimbursements, permitting doctors and hospital administrators to allocate their own resources efficiently, responding to local needs and individual circumstances.

The second program would have replaced the existing Medicaid Early and Periodic Screening, Diagnosis and Treatment Program.

Like the cost containment program, the CHAP legislation is a crucial first step. Other children's health programs also require significant improvement, and the Administration will take steps to meet these needs. But the CHAP program is urgently needed to assure that more low-income children receive regular, high quality primary and preventive care.

In no way was Carter's proposal revolutionary. Moreover, Timothy Stanley (see the quote below) even called it "anemic." However, after decades of stagnation, any breakthrough would have been helpful. And yet,

although Congress was Democratic, the legislation did not pass. In his book *White House Diary*, Carter accuses Ted Kennedy of killing his "sweeping" reform. In 2010, on CBS's *60 Minutes* program, Carter said, "The fact is that we would have had comprehensive health care now, had it not been for Ted Kennedy's deliberately blocking the legislation that I proposed. It was his fault. Ted Kennedy killed the bill." [19]

Carter and Kennedy were adversaries. Actually, Carter said that fighting between liberals was like a scorpion biting itself. However, in such a situation it would be helpful to listen to the other side. Ted Kennedy cannot now defend himself. However, that is what Timothy Stanley, author of *Kennedy vs. Carter: The 1980 Battle for the Democratic Party's Soul* (2010), writes about that conflict:

> Carter should take some of the blame for floating an anemic piece of legislation that, arguably, would have done more harm than good to the cause of health care reform. Kennedy's opposition was principled and rational, and he wasn't just speaking for himself. One interesting difference between then and now is that in the 1970s, the demand for health care reform was tied to a genuine mass movement. Kennedy was just its figurehead and Carter underestimates the senator's influence. Liberalism had more political clout back then, and liberals had enough confidence in their ideas to think they would outlive Carter's moderate administration. They were wrong, but their miscalculation was understandable. [20]

Throughout the 1970s, Ted Kennedy campaigned for national health insurance (NHI) – a single payer, compulsory system open to all. It was much like the "public option" advocated by liberals in 2009-10. Kennedy's fighting was personal: he saw health care reform as his contribution to his family's legacy.

In 1975, Kennedy stopped negotiations with Gerald Ford over a compromise bill. . . . Polls predicted that the Democrats would recapture the presidency in 1976. Why, should they accept a Republican offer? They only had to wait a year and put together their own reform.

Timothy Stanley writes:

> As a presidential candidate in 1976, Carter equivocated on NHI. In

truth, this Southern moderate never liked the idea. A proto-Clinton, he preferred low-cost free-market solutions to public ills. Nonetheless, in order to win over the money and manpower of the UAW [United Auto Workers], Carter endorsed NHI. After his election, he put Great Society architect Joseph Califano (head of Health Education and Welfare) in charge of drawing up legislation. The UAW met with Califano and was shocked when he told them not to expect the support of the president for reform. He eventually quit his job in frustration at stonewalling by Carter.[20]

Under the pressure of liberals, the administration endorsed the Carter's NHI proposal in 1978. President Carter promised reform in three stages. The first stage, and the only one ever defined, addressed hospital cost-containment aiming at deflating medical bills. There was no commitment to comprehensive coverage. Ted Kennedy was shocked: the administration even maintained that any future program be run by private insurers, eliminating any "public option" for consumers to buy directly from the government. Also, this package was likely to increase the price of health care, as doctors would raise their fees to compensate for the loss of revenue.

Were liberals mad to throw away this opportunity for reform, no matter how slight? The polls said not. By 1979, Kennedy was the universal favorite to replace Carter as the Democratic nominee in 1980. Polls put him ahead of both Carter and the Republican candidate Ronald Reagan by margins of 2-1. All Kennedy had to do . . . was enter the primaries, beat Carter, beat Reagan, and then he could push through congress the legislation he wanted.

Ultimately, Ted Kennedy's presidential ambitions were thwarted by historical accident. In late 1979, hostages were seized at the US embassy in Tehran and the USSR invaded Afghanistan. These crises, and the media's revisiting of the Chappaquiddick tragedy, gave Carter a bump in support and helped him win enough early primaries to clinch the nomination. Liberals backed the wrong horse and health care reform didn't resurface as a possibility until 1993.[20]

This probably exonerates Ted Kennedy in his fight with Carter. And yet, having killed the Nixon reform did trouble his conscience "When asked in interviews about his biggest regret as a senator, Kennedy often recalled his failure to make a deal to pass President Nixon's sweeping health care proposal in the early 1970s. Kennedy said that at the time he did not think it went far enough."[21]

But those conflicts, no matter how regrettable, are history now.

Who Cares about Health Care?

In 1981 Carter's miserable presidency was ended by Ronald Reagan. No matter how much he was hated by the left in his lifetime, today all but agree that Reagan was perhaps one of the greatest American presidents, if only because he (not Gorbachev as many believe) defeated the Evil Empire – and that changed the whole world.

As for health care, Reagan was virulently against "socialized" medicine.[22] However, he left his legacy in Medicare.

In 1983, during Congressional debates, the emphasis shifted from improving access to health care to decreasing its cost. A powerful factor that prevented the new legislation from being defeated was the looming Social Security financial crisis. (It is still looming now, even more threateningly.) At that time the status quo was quite gloomy. In 1967, Medicare paid $4.7 billion to 19 million beneficiaries. By 1985, the expenditures had reached $72.3 billion for 31.1 million beneficiaries: a factor of 30 as compared to the increased number of people covered. Social Security was quickly moving to bankruptcy. Congress had to act, forgetting about ideological differences.

President Reagan and a split Congress agreed to a radical new payment scheme for Medicare, which trimmed billions of dollars from the federal budget and greatly reduced medical inflation, yet still maintaining quality of care.

The new payment scheme was simple. Medicare no longer paid hospitals whatever they billed the government (their costs, plus an additional profit margin). Instead, Medicare paid a fixed price linked to each patient's condition or diagnosis-related group (DRG). That price might vary somewhat due to regional adjustments, but it was essentially set in advance (the so-called "prospective payment system" – PPS). The effect of this system was dramatic and immediate. The rate of growth in Medicare hospital payments dropped from 16.2% a year (1980 through 1983) to 6.5% (1987 through 1990). No longer paid to "pad stays," hospitals quickly switched gears. Between 1982 and 1988, Medicare hospital days dropped 20%.[23]

This reform seemed "heretical" to free-marketers. However, Reagan understood that being for "small government" as a *regulator* did not mean abandoning efforts to see that taxpayers got their money's worth from government as *purchaser*. Efficient hospitals made money; inefficient ones lost money. Within that context, DRGs represented deregulation.

Another of Reagan's major achievements must be mentioned here. In July 1988, with bipartisan support, the Medicare Catastrophic Coverage Act was signed into law. The law authorized the most significant expansion of Medicare benefits since its creation in 1965.[24] Among the new benefits was increased coverage of inpatient hospital stays and a revolutionary breakthrough: payment for outpatient prescription drugs, including home IV therapy. Drug co-payments and deductibles were also to be gradually decreased and payment limits established. Regrettably, only 18 months later, Congress and President George H. W. Bush had to completely repeal the law. What happened was that the well-to-do elderly who had protection against catastrophic health situations did not want to pay new taxes to pay for coverage of all the Medicare enrollees.

This was one of the most shameful events in the history of America's health care.

By the end of his presidency Ronald Reagan was suffering from memory decline, which appeared to be the onset of Alzheimer's disease (though the diagnosis was officially announced only in 1994). Since then, he and Nancy became active supporters of stem-cell research that offered a possible cure for Alzheimer's. However, during his presidency and under all the following presidents (including Barack Obama) the issue of long-term health care (together with the accelerating costs of nursing homes) never came to the front burner. (I will discuss this issue in detail in Chapter 4.)

One could not have expected a breakthrough in health care reform during the presidency of George H.W. Bush (1989-1993), and in fact, there was none. However, according to contemporary reporting, Bush used the tax system to "encourage and empower" individuals to buy health insurance.

To help, insurance market reforms were planned that would make it possible for everyone to purchase health insurance, regardless of pre–existing conditions. It actually meant that purchase of health insurance would be mandatory. The cost of coverage would depend on one's income: the poorer one was the less the policy would cost.

No matter how strongly the Republicans today vilify individual mandate, we know that Nixon was the first to explore the idea of individual health care in 1970. Twenty years later, after the extreme conservatism of Ronald Reagan, George H.W. Bush became a surprising supporter of the individual mandate. In his last State of the Union Address in January 1992, he said:

> My plan provides insurance security for all Americans while preserving and increasing the idea of choice. We make basic health insurance affordable for all low-income people not now covered. We do it by providing a health-insurance tax credit of up to $3750 for each low-income family. The middle class gets help, too. And by reforming the health insurance market, my plan assures that Americans will have access to basic health insurance even if they change jobs or develop serious health problem. We must bring costs under control, preserve quality, preserve choice and reduce people's nagging daily worry about

health insurance. My plan, the details of which I will announce shortly, does just that.[25]

However, there was no time left for Bush. On November 3, 1992, Bill Clinton became the 42nd President of the United States.

Health care was on Bill Clinton's agenda from the very first day of his presidency. In January 1993 the Task Force on National Health Care Reform was created, with First Lady Hillary Clinton as its chair. By the fall, a draft of the reform was ready, and on September 22 Clinton delivered a health care address to a joint session of Congress. In it he outlined the core element of the plan: mandating employers to provide health insurance to all employees through strongly regulated health maintenance organizations.

The plan immediately met opposition from conservatives, libertarians, and the health insurance industry. The latter launched a radio, print, and TV advertising campaign called "Harry and Louise." Some readers may still remember it: a suburban forty-something couple is desperate about bureaucratic and other hurdles within the proposed health reform plans and urges viewers to contact their representatives with requests to oppose the reform.

At that time, the legislation was not yet polished; it would be delivered to Congress only on November 20, 1993. However, debates were already in full swing. Here is the health plan's essential features: [26]

> • Each U.S. citizen and permanent resident alien was required to enroll in a qualified health plan and was forbidden to dis-enroll until covered by another plan.
>
> • It listed minimum coverages and maximum annual out-of-pocket expenses for each plan.
>
> • It proposed the establishment of corporate "regional alliances" of health providers to be subject to a fee-for-service schedule.
>
> • People below a certain set income level were to pay nothing.
>
> • Funding was to be sent to the states for the administration of this plan, beginning at $13.5 billion in 1993 and reaching $38.3 billion in 2003.

The history of the struggle for and defeat of Clinton's health care reform is quite dramatic. Detailed time–table of the events is reported in[27].

On September 23rd, the day after Clinton's speech in Congress, the overnight polls showed that the reform had two-thirds approval. Commentators praised Clinton for establishing the right principles that challenged Americans to a

---

historic mission. A.M. Rosenthal wrote in the *New York Times* that "the principle of health coverage for all was an achievement that Clinton could already nail to the wall."

The year 1994 began with the Whitewater scandal that undermined trust in the president. Gradually, one by one, the organizations that had endorsed the reform were backing out. By spring of 1994, the Clinton reform was dead. All attempts to achieve compromises failed.

Paul Starr, one of ten people on the health policy team who had written and re-written the plan, wrote in 1995:

> A year later, almost to the day, Senate Majority Leader George Mitchell pronounced health care reform dead. The funeral was private; no crowds gathered in mourning. While opinion surveys continued to show strong support for the ingredients of reform, the complexity of the plans and onslaught of criticism had even left many supporters bewildered and uncertain. The opposition had focused attention on what those with good health care might lose. Commentators turned on the president. On the eve of the midterm election, Joe Klein told the CBS Evening News audience that the president had led the country into a blind alley with his grandiose reform plan.[28]

Not many know that apart from the Clinton plan, there were other proposals on the table: the Cooper, Chafee, Moynihan, Mitchell, Cooper and Grandy, and some mainstream group plans, which were all defeated. However, as Paul Starr acknowledges:

> It is also a story of strategic miscalculation on the part of the president and those of us who advised him. In 1993, 23 Republican senators, including then Minority Leader Robert Dole, cosponsored a bill introduced by Senator John Chafee that sought to achieve universal coverage through a mandate . . . on individuals to buy insurance. Nearly every major health care interest group had endorsed substantial reforms – grandiose ones, in fact. The American Medical Association (AMA) and Health Insurance Association of America (HIAA), the two great, historic bastions of opposition to compulsory health insurance, both went on record in support of an employer mandate and universal coverage. Even the U.S. Chamber of Commerce endorsed an employer mandate, as did many large corporations. Other groups came out variously for reform options that ran along a spectrum from Canadian-style, single-payer programs on the left to managed competition and medical savings accounts and radical changes in tax policy on the right. Under the circumstances, it was easy to believe the country was ready for substantial reform and that a market-oriented, consumer-

choice approach to universal coverage, positioned in the center, could become a platform for consensus.

It was easy to believe, but it turned out to be wrong.[28]

The Clinton plan is often called the Hillary Clinton plan. The participation of the First Lady in government affairs on such a scale was unique in American history. It even became a constitutional issue, and the Task Force on National Health Care Reform was sued. Hillary won, but the whole health care enterprise, followed by the Clinton sex scandal, cast a dark cloud over her. She needed all her strength and determination to recover, first as a U.S. Senator, and then as a candidate for the presidency.

In his 1995 State of the Union Address Clinton said: Last year we almost came to blows over health care, but we didn't do anything . . .Let's do whatever we have to do to get something done. Let's at least pass meaningful insurance reform."[29] In fact, Congress extended health-care insurance for 5 million children. The end of Clinton's presidency culminated in a budget surplus. Clinton was planning to spend that money on entitlement programs. In 1999 he said: "If we set aside 60% of the surplus for Social Security and 16% for Medicare, over the next 15 years that saving will achieve the lowest level of publicly held debt since right before World War I, in 1917."[30] This did not happen, and now a budget surpus seems like a fairy tale.

During George W. Bush's two terms as a President (2001-2009) no tangible health care reform was launched. There were, however a few important health care issues that he addressed.

Bush believed that one of the most crucial problems of America's health care system that strongly contributed to health care cost was aggressive malpractice litigation against doctors. In 2005 he signed the act that restricted class action suits in state courts. Unfortunately, it was just a palliative. The more general issue is still unresolved and has not been pushed to the front burner by President Obama.

One of Bush's achievements was signing the Medicare Modernization Act that created Medicare D. The Medicare prescription drug program reduces by 16% to 30% prices for most brandname drugs, and by 30% to 60% prices for generics; for low–income seniors a $600 annual subsidy is also provided.[31]

This program, however, is complicated and difficult to understand, especially for some elderly who have to choose a proper option, which is not an easy task. It also has a serious coverage gap, the so-called "Medicare donut hole." "After a Medicare beneficiary surpasses the prescription drug coverage limit, he/she is financially responsible for the entire cost of prescription drugs until the

---

expense reaches the catastrophic coverage threshold."[32]

This hole is supposed to have been closed in the Obama health care legislation.

Another of Bush's achievements was establishing health savings accounts (HSAs)[33]: tax-free accounts that could be used to pay for medical expenses. In order to have more affordable coverage for low-income families that do not have access to employer-sponsored plans, refundable tax credits were established.

To help small business owners and employees, Bush supported creation of Association Health Plans that would allow employers to combine forces to be able to negotiate lower health care primiums. The legislation, the Small Business Health Fairness Act of 2005 (H.R. 525)[34], was passed in the House (263-165) but, for procedural reasons, never came to a vote in the Senate. This is in spite of the fact that, according to Congressional Budget Office estimates, the association health plans could reduce insurance premiums on average by 13%, and decrease the number of uninsured by hundreds of thousands.

Those were Bush's achievements. At the same time he twice ruthlessly vetoed the bipartisan State Children's Health Insurance Program (CHIP) bill, which would have covered millions of American children, not only the poorest, but also a number of middle-class children whose families could not afford necessary medical care. Bush argued that the bill program was expanding socialized medicine. Congress was unable to override the veto.

The 2007-2009 election campaign showed (once again) that a comprehensive health care reform was long overdue and must be implemented. Both Republicans (McCain), and Democrats (competing Hilary Clinton an Barak Obama) proposed their health care plans.

Actually, at that time, some states already began developing their own health care programs. By 2009, three states: Maine, Massachusetts and Vermont, already implemented their own reforms that achieved almost universal coverage of their residents. At that time 14 more states were considering comprehensive reforms.[35]

But now it is history. The *today* is President Obama's brand-new health care reform, *Patient Protection and Affordable Care Act* (usually abbreviated as ACA). I will attempt to review it in a separate chapter.

And now it is time to see how health care systems work in other developed countries.

2. HEALTH CARE IN THE WORLD

> There are nine and sixty ways of
> constructing tribal lays, and every
> single one of them is right.
>
> *Rudyard Kipling*

I would like to begin this chapter with the following quote.

> Of course, there is no single model for national health care systems in
> other countries. Indeed, the differences from country to country are so
> great that the terms "national health care" or "universal coverage" can
> be misleading—as if one collective model shows how other countries
> deal with health care and health insurance. Each country's system is
> the product of its unique conditions, history, politics, and national
> character. Those systems range from the managed competition
> approach of the Netherlands and Switzerland to the more rigid single-
> payer systems of Great Britain, Canada, and Norway, with many
> variations in between.[*]

Which system is "better?" The criteria are quite murky. Is it the cost?
Availability? Wait time? The nation's mortality rate? Or is it "fairness"? In the
concluding chapter I will be comparing "attractiveness" of various health care
system. In this chapter, in describing different systems, I will try to be
objective and reject controversial information as much as possible, especially if
it is politically biased.

In 2000 the World health Organization (WHO) issued the document *World
Health Report 2000. Health Systems: Improving Performance*, which contained
the ranking of 190 countries with respect to their health care systems.[†] This
report is the most detailed and most often cited. Since then "WHO no longer
produces such a ranking table, because of the complexity of the task." France

---

[*] *Comparing Health Care in Canada and the United States and the World*:
http://nextbigfuture.com/2009/08/comparing-healthcase-in-canada-and.html
[†] *WHO 2000 report*: http://www.who.int/whr/2000/en/whr00_en.pdf.

was first on the list; the U.S. was 37th. What brought us down was the categories *Fairness In Financial Contributions*: No54-55, *Health Distribution*: No32, and *Health Performance Level*: No70. What these categories mean, especially the third one, is not quite clear. In *Health Level* we are No24, a bit lower than Germany (No22). At the same time, the category *Responsiveness Level* awards us the No1 rating, while France is No3.[*]

However, there were other rankings. France did not lead them all; but America was inevitably at the bottom. As I mentioned in the Introduction, when this book had already been written, new Bloomberg's ratings were published: The World's Most Efficient Health Care Systems[†], and The World's Healthiest Countries.[‡]

In the health care efficiency ranking, three criteria were used: life expectancy (60% score), relative per capita cost of health care (30%), and absolute per capita cost of health care (10%). In this ranking, the U.S. took 46th place, while Hong Kong took first place.

In the health ranking, the main factors were: life expectancy at birth (10% score); death from diseases (40% of score); death rate by three age groups: less than 14, 15-64 and 65 and up (40% of score); and survival to 65 and life expectancy at 65, gender–ratio weighted (10% of score). The U.S. was ranked 33d, while Singapore was first.

As for France, in these rankings it fell respectively to 19th and 13th place.

The WHO ranking has been criticized for its bias to the left. In the Report's content the U.S., which is accused of social irresponsibility, is kind of a "bad guy." What probably brought America down in Bloomberg's ranking, was, in the health care efficiency: life expectancy (60% score) and relative per capita cost of health care (30%); in the nations' health ranking: death from diseases (40% of score) and death rate by three age groups (40% of score). I will attempt to defend the U.S. where I feel it should be done, stressing our health care's positive features. As for the French system, as we will see, it does look impressive, whereas the British one does not. I will begin, however, with Canada, which, in America, is a designated health care "whipping boy."

---

[*] *WHO Health Care Ranking by Eight Measures*:
http://www.who.int/whr/2000/en/annex01_en.pd
[†] *Bloomberg's The World' Most Efficient Health Care Systems:*
http://www.bloomberg.com/visual-data/best-and-worst/most-efficient-health-care-countries
[‡] *Bloomberg's. The World' Healthiest Countries:*
http://images.businessweek.com/bloomberg/
pdfs/worlds_healthiest_countries_V2.pdf__

Who Cares about Health Care?

Throughout the world, out of some 200 countries, there are only about 40 with well-established and efficiently working health care systems. Almost all those systems were developed during the last century.

Every country's health care system has its own flavor. However, among them there are only four different models[*]:

• The Bismarck Model, created in the 1883 by Otto von Bismarck: Government regulated private insurance funds work mostly through employers. Payment is made through payroll deductions and taxes. Typical examples include France, Germany, Japan, the Netherlands, and Switzerland.

• The Beveridge Model, named after the First Baron William Beveridge the active proponent of public health care who was instrumental in creating Britain's National Health Service in the 1948: It is completely owned and operated by the government and paid for by taxes; there are no bills. Typical examples include Great Britain, Hong Kong, Italy, Spain, and Scandinavia.

• The Douglas Model. named after Tommy Douglas, Prime Minister of Saskatchewan, Canada, and established in 1947: It is known as Medicare and is funded through taxes. Almost all doctors and hospitals are private. Examples include Canada, South Korea, and Taiwan.

• The Out of Pocket Model: Most services are paid out of pocket. This is a Third World model.

As for America, in a peculiar way, its health care system has in it elements of all four models. We are Britain when treating veterans; we are Canada for the elderly on Medicare; we are Germany for Americans who get insurance through their employers; and we are Zambia when we do not have health insurance.

In the table below I compare the rankings of WHO and the Bloomberg's. Aside from the United States, I have selected 6 countries to discuss (bold) from the abridged list below.

Here are the rankings:

---

[*] *Health Care Systems – The Four Basic Models*:
http://www.pbs.org/wgbh/pages/frontline/sickaroundtheworld/countries/models.html ; an excerpt from the book by T .R. Reid, *The Healing of America: A Global Quest for Better, Cheaper, and Fairer Health Care.* Penguin Press, 2009.

Health Care in the World

Country	WHO	Country	BLMBRG H. C. Efficiency	Country	BLMBRG Nation's Health
France	1	Hong Kong	1	Singapore	1
Italy	2	Singapore	2	Italy	2
Spain	7	**Japan**	3	Australia	3
Japan	9	**Israel**	4	Switzerland	4
Norway	11	Spain	5	**Japan**	5
Greece	14	Italy	6	Israel	6
Netherlands	17	Switzerland	9	Netherlands	8
United Kingdom	18	**United Kingdom**	14	**Germany**	10
Switzerland	20	Austria	16	**France**	13
Belgium	21	**Canada**	17	**Canada**	14
Sweden	23	Malaysia	18	Hong Kong	17
Germany	25	**France**	19	**United Kingdom**	21
Israel	28	Finland	23	Finland	22
Morocco	29	Netherlands	25	Denmark	26
Canada	30	**Germany**	30	South Korea	29
Australia	32	Turkey	44	Un. Arab Emirate	30
United States of America	37	**United States of America**	46	**United States of America**	33

As I mentioned, I will begin with Canada, then go on to three Bismarck Model nations (France, Germany and Japan), followed by the National Model's Great Britain. Israel (a hybrid of Bismarck and National Model) will complete the list.

I have attempted to present the most recent statistical data (typically they are two years behind). Please bear in mind that the numbers I came up with are for illustration only, even if the most recent data (which I had been unable to find) would be slightly different. If not specially referenced, they are from the Organization of Economic Cooperation and Development (OECD). The data published in OECD's reviews are the most objective as they are supplied by the nations presented in reviews.

Canada

I begin the tour of health care systems throughout the world with Canada because, as I mentioned in the Introduction (and everybody knows it) in America Canada is a "whipping boy." If they need an argument against a *health-care-for-all* system no matter what kind (for there are many!) they choose Canada to show how bad its system (and, by default, any such system) is.

Most of those accusations are false. I will try to review what the Canadian health care system truly is in as impartial a way as possible.

But first a few words about Canada's administrative structure and population. Canada is a federation of ten provinces (their populations in thousands are in parentheses): Newfoundland and Labrador (512.7), Prince Edward Island (146.1), Nova Scotia (948.7), New Brunswick (756.0), Quebec (8,054.8), Ontario (13,505.9), Manitoba (1,267.0), Saskatchewan (1,080.0), Alberta (3,873.7), British Columbia (4,622.6), and three "territories": Yukon (36.1), Northwest Territories (43.3), and Nunavut (33.7). The total population is slightly less than 35 million, which is less than that of California (38 million), the largest American state.

The political structure of Canada is somewhat unusual for the 21st century. A former British colony, Canada still has strong constitutional ties with Great Britain and is formally a constitutional monarchy. The British Queen (Elizabeth II) is also the Queen of Canada. The executive power is in the hands of the Queen. However, her formal authority over the country is exercised by a Viceroy, or a Governor General, who is appointed by the Queen but on the advice of the Canadian Prime Minister only! There is no term limit for a Governor General: he/she stays "at Her Majesty'pleasure," but the usual term is five years. Because Canada is a bilingual country, English- and French-speaking Governors generally alternate.[*]

Canada's legislature consists of two chambers: the lower House, the House of Commons, and the upper House, the Senate. The lower house's 308 members are directly elected by those eligible to vote. Each member represents a definite electoral district for not more than five years.

As for the Senate's 105 members, they are personally appointed by the Governor General on the advice of the Prime Minister. According to tradition,

---

[*] In 2005, Michaëlle Jean, Quebec's well-known journalist and a native of Haiti, became the first black Governor General of Canada. In 2010 David Johnson became the Governor General of Canada.

both the Governor General and the Senate rarely interfere with the work of the House of Commons (e.g., opposing a bill).

As I mentioned, Canada is a federation. Like the American states, the provinces and territories have significant independence in dealing with local issues. The federal government does not interfere with the local authorities unless they violate the constitution, which rarely happens. As for the Canada's health care it is governed by individual provinces and territories.

If one goes to Google and types in *medicare*, apart from information on American Medicare, one will find links to similar systems in a few other countries, including Canada. Thus, health care in Canada (which is a target of severe criticism not only in the U.S. but in Canada as well) is Medicare, though this name is unofficial.

Canadian Medicare was born in 1947 in the province of Saskatchewan.[1] Its Premier, Tommy Douglas (who is remembered in Canada as the father of Medicare), introduced and passed the *Saskatchewan Hospitalization Act* that made health care free for the majority of the population. In 1950 Alberta passed a similar program. Ten years later, a national hospital insurance program was introduced. Officially, Medicare was established in Saskatchewan as the first public program in 1962. During the following two decades, a national universal health care system was being developed, culminating in 1984 in the *Canada Health Act*, unanimously passed by both houses of Parliament.

Let me share the following passionate quote.[*][2]

> . . . the movement toward universal health care in Canada started in 1916 (depending on when you start counting), and took until 1962 for passage of both hospital and doctor care in a single province. It took another decade for the rest of the country to catch on. That is about 50 years all together. It wasn't like we sat down over afternoon tea and crumpets and said please pass the health care bill so we can sign it and get on with the day. We fought, we threatened, the doctors went on strike, refused patients, people held rallies and signed petitions for and against it, burned effigies of government leaders, hissed, jeered, and booed at the doctors or the Premier depending on whose side they were on. In a nutshell, we weren't the stereotypical nice polite Canadians. Although there was plenty of resistance, now you could more easily take away Christmas than Health Care, despite the rhetoric that you

---

[*] From a talk given by Karen S. Palmer MPH, MS in San Francisco at the Spring 1999 PNHP (Physicians for National Health Program) meeting.

may hear to the contrary.

And now let us see what Canadian Medicare is all about.

The *Canada Health Act* is the foundation of the entire Health Care system. It is based on five principles[3]:

- Comprehensiveness: All necessary health services, including hospitals, physicians and surgical dentists, must be insured.

- Universality: All insured residents are entitled to the same level of Health Care.

- Portability: Residents who move to a different province or territory are still entitled to coverage from their home province during a minimum waiting period. This also applies to residents who leave the country.

- Accessibility: All insured persons have reasonable access to Health Care facilities. In addition, all physicians, hospitals, etc., must be provided reasonable compensation for the services they provide.

- Provincial Health Insurance: Health insurance in Canada is handled by individual provinces and territories.

Actually, there is no such thing as a "Canadian Health Care System." It is, rather, a conglomerate of provincial systems. They vary, though they have federal guidelines. Each province issues its own Health Card, which is the only document that is requested when one is attended by medical professionals. The benefits provided upon producing a Health Card are guaranteed only to the *public* component of health care.

Who pays for universal health care in Canada? Seventy-five percent of health care costs in Canada are paid by federal and provincial governments. Since the government does not make money (though it prints it!), the money's only source is taxes. Like the U.S., Canada has a progressive tax-bracket–based system. Canadians pay: federal taxes (0-29%), provincial taxes (0-24%), payroll Canada Pension Plan tax (4.95%), Federal Social Security Tax (1.73%), Provincial Employment Tax (0-2%), as well as VAT (Value Added Tax) and sales taxes. [4] My friends, who live in Ontario, told me that from an average middle-class annual salary of $80,000-$90,000,[*] 40% to 50% goes to taxes. In 2004, in Ontario, a special "health premium" (they do not call it a tax) was

---

[*] Whenever sources give expenditures in Canada in dollars, it is most probably Canadian dollars. As of May, 2014 the rate is $1Can = $0.92 US. A while ago the Canadian dollar was significantly weaker.

additionally introduced to patch some holes in financing. As a tax, it is minuscule (at least by American standards). It is progressive, the maximum payment being $900 per year for those earning over $200,000. Of course, private health insurance that would complement "public" coverage is extra. This is a lot; however Canadians also get a lot for their money.

One third of the federal funds withheld through taxes is slated for health care and is distributed among the provinces and territories, complementing their own health care budgets. And that is where the federal government's functions end. The provinces administer the public components of health care (what is covered and how coverage differs from province to province) locally.

In Canada federal and provincial governments pay for all *public* health care required by the *Canada Health Act* from hospital stays (typically, four people in a ward), visits to internists and specialists, and all tests and "necessary procedures.*"

In Canada, among the issues that are only partially in the public domain are vision care (though regular check-ups for children and the elderly are covered), dental care, mental health, cosmetic surgery, orthopedic devices, physical therapy, and long-term care, to name just a few. Most of those services are paid for either through supplemental health insurance, subsidized by employers, or from one's own pocket. One also has to pay for some "extras," such as a hospital room for two people. Dental care is expensive. Those who cannot afford dental insurance (some 17% of the population hesitate to see a dentist, which eventually results in poor general health). Strange as it may seem, in Ontario, one also pays for the use of an ambulance a fee of $54.

The main components of out-of-pocket spending in 2010 were: dental care (20%), nonhospital institutions (mainly long-term care homes) (20%), prescription drugs (17%), vision care (12%), and over-the-counter medications (10%).[5]

Where the necessary treatment or service goes beyond the public domain, the regulations of various provinces are inconsistent. For instance, services of non-physicians who work outside hospitals in some provinces may not be covered. What and how much is not covered from public funds depends on specific situations. Eligibility for extension of public funding may depend on age (children, seniors), income, enrollment in special programs for home care, or diagnosis (e.g., HIV/AIDS, cancer, cystic fibrosis).

Over half of Canadian doctors are internists. The army of 30,000 primary care

---

* Our Medicare pays only 80% of approved costs. As I discuss in the two last chapters, it is good.

physicians is the backbone of the Canadian system: they provide both basic medical treatments and preventive care. As with American HMOs, a visit to a specialist requires a referral by a family physician. Currently in Canada there are 28,000 specialty doctors.

Like the U.S., Canada's health care system does not cover "outpatient" prescription drugs, though drugs administered in hospitals are paid for from public funds. Provinces have programs that help seniors, the poor, and in some cases cover those with special health care issues, like extended dental care, long term services, etc.[*] For example, a combination of private and public funds in Québec achieved universal drug coverage. There is, however, no national program. Two-thirds of Canadians purchase drugs through insurance companies or through their employers. Like the U.S., a significant part of the Canadian population is not fully covered by any program for purchasing medications. Prescription drugs are a high burden on Canadians' budgets: the expenses are about 17.5% of their incomes, and over 20% of sick Canadians do not fill prescriptions.[6]

In the U.S., the cost of drugs is 20% higher than in Canada. In 2012, Canadians spent $752 on drugs per capita whereas American paid $987 (see the table in the concluding chapter). This is in spite of the fact that Canadians consume more drugs than Americans: 12 prescriptions per year, compared with 10.6 prescriptions in America. Many Americans (especially seniors) prefer to purchase drugs in Canada, giving Canadian pharmacies 1 billion U.S. dollars per year!

Why are prescription drugs less expensive in Canada? There are a few reasons for the drug cost disparity.

The main reason is that the cost of patented drugs in Canada is 35 to 45% lower than in the U.S., partly because patent protection in Canada is more limited than in the U.S. Therefore generic drugs appear on the market earlier (although they are relatively more expensive). In the U.S. patents may be extended to allow more profit to cover the development costs.

Provincial governments buy drugs in bulk, thus lowering prices, whereas in the U.S. negotiating drug prices by Medicare is explicitly prohibited. Drug price

---

[*] In Ontario, after the age of 65, all drugs prescribed by a doctor are free. As my Ontario friend has noticed with humor, her mother-in-law had successfully "used up" all her family funds paid as taxes: she had had a few surgeries, an amputation, rehabilitation, and now has free drugs and free transportation once a week to drawing lessons! Well, that is exactly what the elderly eligible for Medicaid have in the U.S. Alas, not for Medicare!

negotiation by insurers is based on evaluation of drug effectiveness. The Canadian Patented Medicine Prices Review Board sets "fair and reasonable prices" on patented drugs, in comparison with similar drugs on the market or average prices in seven OECD nations.

One can see that with respect to prescription drugs the Canadian and U.S. health care systems are not that different. The difference is in how they are administered. The disparities in drug costs could be easily eliminated. Of course, as in many aspects of American life, ideology often dominates and suppresses both reason and economic necessity.

As I already mentioned, in contrast to what is usually claimed by critics, the Canadian health care system is not a centralized, government-directed one. It was not created by government decree: it emerged as a result of initiatives by provinces. It is a conglomerate of public and private services. According to estimates of the Canadian Medical Association, "75 per cent of health-care services are delivered privately, but funded publicly."[7] In 2011, out of approximately $161 billion spent on health care ($4,666 per person), the government spent over $114.5 billion (71%) on public health care, whereas private health care cost the Canadian economy $46.5 billion.[8]

All Canadian hospitals are non-profit and controlled by provincial governments, whereas everyday health care (general practitioners, specialists, chemical labs, and many other services) are private for-profit enterprises. Like in the U.S., physicians join small associations sharing office space, ancillary medical personnel, and necessary services. Doctors' offices, though private and independent, are incorporated into public health care because doctors' bills are typically paid from public funds. Of course they are also opened for services paid by supplemental private insurers.

The Canadian Health Coalition (a liberal lobby group) argues that for-profit clinics are an impediment to the original ideological foundation of public health care: "The proliferation of investor-owned private, for-profit clinics and facilities acts like a viral infection in the body of Canada's public health-care system." However, the network of private services widens, and the symbiosis of private and public health care institutions seems to be practically viable and healthy.

Maternity/paternity leave.[9] The laws may differ from province to province. Typically, the benefits are as follows.

New mothers and fathers are eligible for paid leave through Employment Insurance (EI) program (which also provides unemployment benefits). Both biological and surrogate mothers are entitled to 15 weeks of partly paid maternity leave (irrespective of whether one or more babies were born or adopted): up to 8 weeks before and the rest after the delivery*. They are paid about 55% of "average insurable weekly earning," up to a maximum, which was (in 2012) $485/week. Parents of a new baby can have between them additional 35 weeks of unpaid leave. After parental leave is over, the employer has to provide the same or equivalent job with the same pay.

Employment Insurance, which is financed from payroll deduction by employer of 1.83% worker's salary, up to a maximum amount of $840, pays for paternity leave only if a mother/father has accumulated more that 600 hours of "insurable employment;" and some specific criteria are met. Thus, the benefits are not automatic, and have to be approved. There is also a two-week waiting period before the first paycheck has been issued. Low-income family receives a "Family Supplement."

Let me now turn to an issue that is of acute concern in the U.S. but not in Canada: kindergartens. In Canada they are all private, widely available, and relatively inexpensive: some cost $700/month. For low-income people there are subsidies. There is a more expensive network of home kindergartens for fewer than 10 children.

And now another acute problem both in Canada and America: long-term health (LTH) care. Long-term care is not publicly insured under the *Canada Health Act*. As Canadians say, the "universality" of their health care "**ends at the doors of nursing homes.**"[10]

For a long time Canada has been in denial over the problem of the growing elderly population. Unlike America, which has developed a network of long-term health care facilities from assisted living complexes to nursing homes (albeit many are extremely expensive), in Canada, even finding such a facility is a problem.

Government-subsidized nursing homes are rarities. They are outdated and overcrowded, the waiting time to get a bed can be as long as three to four years, there is no choice of location, and services may be restricted. Also, an annual assessment of the financial situation of the patient's family decides how much of the cost is subsidized, and even then, in addition to the subsidy, some $750 to $1,500 per month must be paid by the elderly and his/her family.[11]

A network of private nursing homes has begun developing only recently. They are expensive by Canadian standards: $40,000 to $70,000 a year ($100 to $200

---

* A comment of my Canadian friend: "Many expecting mothers keep working till the very last days before delivery, thus saving more leave time for later:"

per day). This is significantly less expensive than even non-profit nursing homes in America (over $300 per day). And yet, like in America, this is a very heavy burden on the elderly and his/her family.

One can purchase a private LTH insurance. Only a handful of companies offer such policies, although their number is increasing. Insurance covers LTH care both at home and at a facility, for as long as it is needed. People between 30 and 80 years old can apply for a policy. Depending on the level of benefits, the insurers pay up to $300 per day – tax-free! [10]

This is more generous than in the U.S. (I will discuss our long-term health issues in the last chapter).*

We have learned a lot about Canadian health care. Most people in America believe that it is *worse* than America's. Let us see what the arguments are for and against that belief.

Although it may seem that the American and Canadian systems are not that much different: Both are combinations of one payer (in the U.S. – Medicaid and Medicare), and private systems (in Canada – private doctors' offices and such services as dental insurance and long-term care), however, the roles of those two components are different in each country. For opponents, the most infuriating feature of Canadian health care is its "single-payerness." But this is mostly an ideological argument.

When it comes to the Canadian system's drawbacks, the arguments become serious. The main issue, which is also the major argument against Canada's system, is wait time. It cannot be denied that the wait time in Canada is, on average, higher than in America, and some people have to travel to the U.S. for urgent surgery.† The data on "median wait time" (half of people wait less) are contradictory depending on whether they originate from conservative or liberal sources. I always prefer official data.

The most recent (2008 and 2010) Canadian Federal Reports give the following median wait times: for non-emergency surgeries – 4.3 weeks (with 82.2% waiting less than 3 months.); for MRI and CAT scans – two weeks (with 89.5% waiting less than 3 months); to see a specialist – a little over

---

* Unfortunately, I have been unable to find on the Internet even a single quote for a private long-term insurance policy. Like in the U.S., in order to have a quote one has to enter personal information.

† Canadians "do not come to the US for health care: 99.39%; come for elective care: 0.5%; use the US for emergency care: 0.11%" (Aaron E. Carroll, from: AARP, April 16, 2012 , *5 Myths About Canada's Health Care System*:
http://www.aarp.org/politics-society/government-elections/info-03-2012/myths-canada-health-care.html).

four weeks (with 86.4% waiting less than 3 months).[12]

A 2010 Commonwealth Alliance's survey[13] found that 42% of Canadians responding said that they waited 2 hours or more in the emergency room, vs. 29% of respondents in the U.S.; 43% of Canadians waited 4 weeks or more to see a specialist, whereas in the U.S. it was only 10%. Of course wait time is prioritized. An appendectomy is performed within hours, as is an urgent coronary bypass, angioplasty, or the setting of a broken leg. The most drastic wait time is not an inherent quality of the public system (although bureaucracy does play its role!) but is rather the direct consequence of the shortage of specialists (possibly also operating rooms where a surgeon works), and the scarcity of high-tech diagnostic equipment such as MRI and CT scan machines.* Canada has the same number of doctors per capita as the United States: 2.4/1000 population (2011).[8] However, the number of specialists compared to internists is lower than in the U.S.† Besides, there is a brain drain:‡ the young and talented (especially among specialists) drift to the U.S. where they can earn much more.

As for the second cause (shortage of diagnostic equipment and hospital facilities for special procedures), in my (layman's!) view, the issue is more complex and difficult. Such equipment is located mostly in hospitals, which means that the hospitals have purchased them. And purchased from a provisional government's budget, for all hospitals are non-profit and subsidized by the provisional governments. In contrast, in Boston's North Shore, where I live, there are at least *six* MRI machines (in for profit clinics)! For-profit clinics or hospitals can afford expensive equipment. A government obviously cannot.

This is a serious issue. However, as I have learned from numerous Internet sources, the Canadian government spends millions of dollars attempting to cut the wait time, first of all by injecting money into government-subsidized hospitals and clinics in order to remove the obstacles.

Apart from the wait time, there are other issues that should be analyzed if one wants to understand the difference between the Canadian and American health care systems.

Now we turn to objective statistics, comparing life expectancy, infant mortality

---

* France has fewer MRI and CT scan machines, but more patients use them (see Conclusion).
† In rural areas or small towns, there is also a shortage of internists. This is typical of America also.
‡ The situation is getting better: "For the first time in at least 30 years, more doctors are coming back to Canada than leaving." CTV News, 14 Dec. 2010.
http://www.ctv.ca/CTVNews/CTVNewsAtl1/20050825/doctors_brain_drain_050824/

and obesity. (See a more detailed table at the concluding chapter).

	U.S.A.	Canada
Infant mortality/1000 live births	6.1	5.1
Obesity rate %: female/male	35.5/32.2	32.2/25.2
HC spending as % of GDP	17.6	11.4

The numbers on lower life expectancy and higher infant mortality in the U.S. can be found on quite a few websites as an evidence of inferiority of American health care.

The source from which the following quote has been borrowed [14] draws a more objective picture. Why do Canadians live longer?

> One reason is due to the excess number of accidents and homicides in the U.S. compared to Canada. In fact 50%-85% of the mortality gap between American and Canadian adults in their twenties can be explained by the increased American accident/homicide rates. For people over 50, 30%-50% of the difference in age-specific mortality rates can be attributed to the excess number of heart disease patients in the U.S. These heart disease findings are more likely driven by American lifestyle choices rather than the efficacy of the U.S. medical system.

But that does not explain everything. As the statistics show, the difference in mortality rates between the two countries may also be the result of the more diverse ethnic/racial composition of the American population: the mortality of Caucasians in both countries is virtually the same. Thus, it is tempting to claim that the difference has nothing to do with the inferiority of the American system, but rather results from the higher mortality (for various reasons) of the non-Caucasian population. However, when the ethnic/race identifier has been dropped and the correlation of mortality with affluence/poverty is considered, the key to the situation becomes obvious.

Because the Canadian egalitarian system does not distinguish between the rich and the poor – everybody is eligible for the same high quality health care (with insignificant "ripples" to do with access of the more affluent to non-public medicine) – the mortality rate is more uniform through various strata of the population. (There is, however, variation among various provinces/territories, and mortality among, for example, the Inuits, is higher because health care is less accessible there.) Therefore the "poor" do not die more often than the "rich."

As for the first ethnic/race argument: to think of it, it does converge with the affluence/poverty argument. The non-Caucasian minorities in America are less (too often much less) affluent, and their access to the market health care is restricted (unless they are below poverty level, and then they are eligible for Medicaid, which would not cost them a penny).

The cultural differences also matter: low-educated low-income people either do not have access to information on the harmful aspects of their life style (consumption of unhealthy food, smoking, etc.) or ignore it.* And do not forget the American elderly. No matter what the opponents claim. Medicare, the foundation of health care for millions of American elderly, covers only 80% of health care costs. Living on a Social Security check to pay the remaining 20% (plus the deductibles and co-payments) may be difficult if not impossible. Only those on Medicaid are equivalent to the Canadian elderly.

The second serious issue is infant mortality. In its database [15] CIA places the U.S. somewhere between Cuba (5.74/1000 births) and Belarus (6.34). All CIA's numbers are slightly higher than the ones in the table above, but basically, their information is correct. Is America's higher infant mortality a result of its "inferior" health care? The answer in most cases is NO, although there are a few factors that need to be considered.

Doctors know that a significant predictor of infant mortality is a baby's birth weight:

> In fact U.S. infant mortality is lower for low birth weight babies than Canadian infant mortality for low birth weight babies. Overall infant mortality, however, is higher in the U.S. because the incidence of babies with low birth weight is higher than in Canada. This may be due to demographic or epidemiological factors, or it may be the case that the U.S. is better at having a live birth for a low birth weight baby. [14]

The last argument is important. American doctors fight for the lives of babies no matter how small, under-carried, or even birth-defected. Those efforts are unprecedented. As a result, the number of such babies born in the U.S. is higher than in Canada (and quite possibly anywhere in the world). And this is in spite of the fact that their survivability is lower than that of regular birth weight babies. Hence the "bad" statistics placing America close to Belarus.

One can see from the table that obesity in America is much higher than in Canada (especially among men). I am not going to discuss this issue: it is on the frontline of the American media, talk-shows, etc. There are at least two

---

* Having said that, it does not mean that ethnic/racial genetic predispositions contributing to early death can be ignored.

factors significantly contributing to this dramatic situation: eating unhealthy food and a life-style that discourages physical activity. The most dramatic (if not tragic) fact is that our children are sliding into that abyss more and more. Our health care system does not bear much responsibility for that situation. America is a free country, and nobody can force people to change their habits. People need to understand the danger.* Whether America will have more "public" health care or not, obesity, and diabetes as its almost inevitable consequence, will remain a danger of an existential scale.

An important issue still to be discussed is access to medical care in Canada as compared to that in the U.S. The efficiency of the Canadian and U.S. systems may not differ much. Access to internists in Canada is as easy as it is in the U.S. As I mentioned, due to the insufficient number of specialty doctors, the wait time to see one may be higher than in the U.S. And here are some interesting facts:

Canada in general has a lower disease incidence rate, but treatment rates are generally higher in the U.S. Further, these differences decrease even more if we look only at Caucasians in each country. However, "In Canada, the main reason for an unmet need was because the wait was too long or the treatment was unavailable. . . . In the U.S. most people who do not receive treatment fail to do so because of cost considerations."[14]

Before Obamacare, not many American health care plans covered annual physical examination. However, when it comes to high-risk illnesses, the preventive services in America are better than in Canada:[14]

> • *Mammograms*: 88.6% of American females 40-69 have had a mammogram compared to 72.3% of Canadians.
> • *PAP smear*: 86.3% of American females 20-69 had a PAP smear in the last 3 years compared to 75.1% of Canadians.
> • *Prostate screening*: 54.2% of American men 40-69 have had a PSA test compared to 16.4% of Canadians.

The author of the quoted article attributes the above differences to *moral hazard*:

> Canadians know that if they get a disease their government will pay for their care. Thus, they may be less motivated to ask for preventive services. . . . Further, most [American] patients strongly wish to avoid disease, not simply due to cost considerations, but because of the

---

* When traveling to Japan, we will see that a person with the onset of obesity receives a warning from the health care authority.

physical and mental impact the disease would have on their life.[14]

And now the *malpractice insurance* hazard. Though, as Canadian sources claim, malpractice suits plague Canada, the situation is not as bad as in the U.S. The difference in the extra cost due to these expenses reflects the difference in how health care is administered in both countries. I will be discussing the malpractice litigation problem in the U.S. in the penultimate chapter. Here, suffice it to say that in Canada "the total cost of settlements, legal fees, and insurance comes to $4 per person each year, but in the United States it is $16."[16] In the U.S., the cost of malpractice insurance to doctors is threatening to kill the medical profession. In Canada, it does not appear to be as detrimental.

A few words about health care administrative costs in Canada and the U.S. The estimate of administrative overheads in the Internet are contradictory: the Canadian numbers are low and impressive, whereas the American sources drastically increase those numbers.

The American Medical Association (AMA) study (2010)[17] indicates that "hidden administrative costs dwarfed monetary expenditures, concluding that true administrative costs are many times higher in Canada than in the United States."

However, another study[18] reports that the amount of time American doctors and nurses spend interacting with insurance companies is four times greater than in Canada, thus significantly contributing to administrative costs.

As a layman who lives in the U.S., I would rather believe the second study. Besides, the AMA's arguments have strong ideological overtones: AMA has always been against "health care for all."

To summarize the comparison of the health care systems in Canada and the U.S.: It seems that although Americans have higher rates of diabetes, arthritis, chronic lung disease, high blood pressure and obesity (all of these issues may be a direct consequence of lifestyle), success of treatment, especially of breast cancer, is higher in the U.S. (largely because of the timely administration of diagnosis and treatment). Health care is much more expensive in America than in Canada. Both Canadians and Americans have access to high quality health care, though Canadians spend about 55% of what Americans do. In Canada, individuals and insurance companies spend between $4,890 (Québec) and $6,070 (Alberta) on health care annually; this includes "non-public" spending on eye and dental care and drugs. And the government expenses in the U.S. are also higher than those in Canada. Although they mostly cover and subsidize just a few programs,* but the numbers of Americans depending on the government subsidies is enormous. I will discuss this issue in the concluding chapter. Canadian system provides affordable health care for all, and therefore is "fair." However, it has serious drawbacks. Even exercising "fairness" one encounters an eternal compromise: give and take. The Canadian systeseems to have found a reasonable compromise. Its drawbacks are treatable. Eventually, a more constructive symbiosis between the public and private approach will be developed in Canada.

France

France has always been in the heart of Europe, and not merely geographically. The French Revolution (1789–1799), proclaiming *liberty, equality, and fraternity*, caused a social upheaval that changed Europe forever. The guillotine, a device that made revolutionary terror extremely efficient, plunged France into a blood bath. However, the *Declaration of the Rights of Man and of the Citizen* that came out of it has become a foundation of Western democracy. In spite of his defeat, Napoleon Bonaparte, who turned the first European republic into an empire and bloodied the continent at the same time, completed Europe's transformation.

The mottos of the Revolution are still an essential part of the French understanding of themselves and the world. Equality, pluralism, and solidarity are the foundations of the French health care system.

Today France is a "unitary semi-presidential republic." Its population of 65 million is the second largest in Europe after Germany and it also has nine overseas territories (former colonies). France has the fifth largest world economy, is a full-fledged nuclear power, and has the third largest stockpile of nuclear weapons in the world. Eighty percent of its electricity is supplied by nuclear power plants.

A decade ago France had the best educational system in the world (unfortunately there are signs of its declining). And, as I already mentioned, in 2000, the World Health Organization (WHO) placed France first in its rating of

---

* The U.S. government directly pays only for Medicaid, the State Children's Health Insurance Program (CHIP), the Veterans Administration, and Military Health Care. It also subsidizes Medicare, although Americans pay a special Social Security tax, FICA, a part of which goes to Medicare payments for the elderly.

the world's health care systems. However, according to the most recent Bloomberg's ratings, France has lost its first place. Today France is in the throes of a severe economic crisis, at the heart of which is its Social Security System, with health care being just one of many headaches.

In this world of uncertainty and crisis, France has created a safety net for its population, including those who are not legal citizens.[1]

Until recently, the retirement age in France was 60, and in some cases even 58. In October 2010, in spite of violent demonstrations, the French Senate raised the retirement age to 62.

Paid vacations seem enormous to Americans. For example, Stephany Marchand, a senior journalist, has eight weeks of vacation. "Eight weeks, yes. I know it may be surprising for you because I know in the U.S. you might have only two or three, if you're lucky, but we have eight."[2]

Like most Frenchmen, Marchand has no guilt about taking so much time off. In fact, *it's the law: full-time workers in France are guaranteed at least five weeks vacation* – guaranteed those long lazy days in the sun, and leisurely lunches in outdoor cafes.

On top of the five weeks, there are another dozen public holidays, and a maximum 35-hour workweek, with no paid overtime allowed. Managers like Marchand, who work more than 35 hours a week, get more time off. "The so-called 35-hour work week gives us 22 more days a year," says Marchand.

To an outsider, France seems to live in an economically different world. The near 10% unemployment rate in France is normal, whereas it would be a disaster for American economy. Generous unemployment benefits often discourage people from finding new jobs. Partly because of these benefits, France's economy, even in good times, is not burgeoning, although it has emerged from the 2008-2009 recession faster than other European countries. On the positive side, the French are not suffering from credit card debt the way we Americans are because they use mostly debit cards. They have 39 million debit cards and just 9 million credit cards.[3]

Now let me turn to health care. In America, when we talk about the French health care system we blame it for being "socialistic." However, the French detest and reject that notion, claiming that it is in Canada and Britain where medicine is socialized whereas theirs is not. Having achieved universal coverage, they have not sacrificed their right to choose physicians, hospitals, and treatment as we, Americans believe must be. They have simply found a rational way of maintaining it. As a result, in France there are no uninsured, and the system has developed a health care safety net for all.

Comparing the French system with ours, one can immediately see a common feature. Their system is a kind of Medicare (and a better Medicare than in Canada). The difference is that in the U.S., Medicare covers only the elderly, whereas in France it has expanded to serve the entire population.

> In France, the sicker you get, the less you pay. Chronic diseases, such as diabetes, and critical surgeries, such as a coronary bypass, are reimbursed at 100%. Cancer patients are treated free of charge. Patients suffering from colon cancer, for instance, can receive Genentech's Avastin without charge. In the U.S., a patient may pay $48,000 a year.

> Everyone has access to the same basic coverage through national insurance funds, to which every employer and employee contribute. The government picks up the tab for the unemployed who cannot gain coverage through a family member.[4]

There is one major ideological factor that distinguishes the two systems. The French believe that in order for the nation to be healthy *the healthy should pay for care of the sick*. This belief is nationwide, shared by both the left and the right of the political spectrum. In a survey posing the question, "Should the healthy pay for the sick or should everyone get back only what they put into the system?" 86% of the people responded "yes" and 95% approved of mandatory insurance.[5]

The commitment to universal health coverage in France is based on the principle of solidarity: there should be mutual aid and cooperation between sick and healthy, and that health insurance payroll taxes should depend on the ability to pay, not economic risk.

To the French, all such "unusual" features like "the sicker you get, the less you pay"[*] are the manifestations of solidarity, rather than "socialism." Incomprehensible as it may sound to Americans, the word "solidarity" signifies to the French an important social concept, and not only in health care. The French counterpart of our Department of Health and Human Services is the Ministry of Health and Solidarity. French businesses also pay a special Corporate Social Solidarity Contribution Fee financing protection of the self-employed.

Before I go into details, one note: In 2004, France underwent health care

---

[*] An example: In the list below of what is covered and how, you will see that a hospital stay greater than 30 days is 100% covered, rather than 80% if the illness is less severe.

reform that slightly tightened everybody's belts. However, because (and unfortunately) too often websites do not tell you when they were put on the Internet or modified, some data I came across were outdated, and needed to be checked. If a reader wants to learn more and explore the Internet in more details, this should be kept in mind.[6]

French National Health Insurance currently faces a severe financial crisis. The deficit is now close to €21 billion ($27 billion[*]) and is estimated to increase to $90 billion by the end of the year 2020.[7] The primary objective of the recent health care reform was to lower costs.

Among measures to do that is restriction of patients' ability to choose doctors they like because of gate-keeping by primary care physicians. The French resist this measure even though they have a lesser reimbursement should they refuse to go through that gate. Strange as it may seem, in spite of the rise of health care costs, France isn't likely to make major changes to the system most citizens say they like. "Why would they?" says Shanny Peer, policy director at the independent French-American Foundation: "France gets better results for less money and everyone is covered."[4]

The foundations of the French health care system were mostly laid in the 1930s. The original system was very much like American Medicare, with the difference that it covered all salaried workers rather than only the elderly. White collar and agricultural workers were not originally covered.

The 1930s reforms were driven forward by unions against doctors' resistance. Eventually, a compromise was reached establishing a "medical chart" that satisfied doctors. It guaranteed fee for service and free choice of doctors by patients. Doctors were allowed to set their fees, and – quite an unusual feature – patients had to pay doctors directly and received reimbursement later. The system was funded from payroll deductions.[†] These principles remain intact today.

In 1940, within just six weeks, a larger and better equipped French army was defeated by the Nazis. France was occupied. The southern half of the country remained what was called a semi-independent republic, the so-called Vichy state. However, the Vichy state was far from independent. Actually, it collaborated with the Germans, even actively supporting rounding up and

---

[*] € is the symbol of the single European currency, the Euro, accepted by 17 of 27 countries of the European Union. The value of 1€ varies, and as of May 2014, it corresponds approximately to $1.36. I will be indicating all monetary units in U.S. dollars.

[†] In the US, the AMA adamantly opposed such a feature until the creation of Medicare in 1965.

extraditing the Jews.[8] Health care was in turmoil.

Meanwhile, the exiled Free French groups in England were planning future reforms. In 1945, right after the end of the war, a government body, Securité Sociale (Social Security), was created. Its task was to resurrect the health care system. Doctors' private practice and the fee-for-service system were re-established.

In the new France the powerful pre-war forces, such as employers and mutual aid societies, mostly lost their influence because they had collaborated with the Nazis. The unions were clear, as were the doctors, for they had not collaborated.[*] They became the main force behind the reforms. This is the system that was created on the ruins of WWII:

> Doctors resisted payment by third parties, and patients paid the bill and then sought reimbursement from Securité Sociale. . . . Even today, patients, except in expensive procedures, pay the doctor directly and get reimbursement from the plan. The fee schedule was to be set and the Securité Sociale payment would be 80% of the fee, just as [American] Medicare was expected to pay only 80%.[9]

As could have been expected, the government fee schedule met doctors' resistance. It took quite a while before doctors accepted it. In 1960 President of France General De Gaulle himself intervened. He said: "I saved France on a colonel's salary!" The doctors gave in.

Today the French health care system is one of the most expensive in the world (11.6% of the GDP, after the Netherlands, 12.0%, and the U.S., 17.7%[10]). Its funding is extremely complex and difficult to comprehend. Information on the Internet is often controversial, vague and even incorrect. It took me hours to understand even the basics of what the French pay for their health care.

To begin with, Michael Moore's insistence in his controversial movie *Sicko* that Americans pay more taxes than French and most of Europe is wrong: The French pay in taxes and payroll deductions more than Americans do. However, "paying more" is not a simple concept. Paying more for what? If we want to understand the French system, we must compare apples with apples. If we do it right, then *we, the people*, will be able to decide if the French lesson is worth learning.

First, let me share with you what I have learned and understood about how

---

[*] For example, doctors often treated wounded Resistance fighters in spite of the threat of death.

French health care is funded (although I might have not grasped everything). I will be discussing what the French buy for that money later.

Unlike the U.S. and many other countries, the French tax system is extremely complex (I have even come across words that describe it as "threateningly complex!"). It is a combination of payroll deductions (they do not even call them "taxes") that people see on their slips when they get paid (wages or pensions), and income taxes that they pay once a year, or if they prefer, in installments.

Benefits	Rate Employee	Rate Employer
Health Insurance	0.75%	12.8%
Accidents at Work		3%
Family Benefits		5.4%
General Social Contribution (CSG)	7.5% – wages 6.6% – pensions 8.2% – investments	
Social Debt Repayment (CRDS)	0.5%	
Unemployment monthly ceiling: $15,000	2.4%	4.4%
Main Pension	6.75%	9.9%
Supplementary Pension. wages up to $3,750/month wages $3,750 to $11,250/month	3% 8%	4.5% 12%
TOTAL without supplementary pension with supplementary pension	17.9% 24%	35.5% 45%

In funding health care, employers' contributions are absolutely crucial. And there is no single national insurance charge, like in Canada or England. Even as payroll deductions, different components of funding are charged separately.

In the table above, the most important deductions (as percentages of wages) that the French paid in 2010 are shown.[11]

The CSG deduction depends on the income source. In adding up the numbers, I took 7.5% deducted from wages only. It is interesting to note that the French pay a special levy on mandatory social debt repayment (CRDS). Shouldn't we Americans take care of that in our taxes?

After 2010, the French became eligible for a Social Security pension after the age of 62. There are "basic" and "supplemental" pensions. Both are compulsory, though paid from different funds. The basic pension depends only on the number of years/quarters that the employee has worked. The deductions for supplemental pensions depend on the wage bracket. To arrive at reasonable numbers, I arbitrarily averaged the employee's and employer's deductions as 6.1% and 9.5%

There are additional deductions. Among them is the 3.4% "Additional Social Levy" (abbreviated PS) on employees, or 0.16% "Corporate Social Solidarity Contribution" on employers to finance social protection of the self-employed, which I have already mentioned.

But what about income taxes? They are progressive and substantial. The wages up to $7,975 are not taxable. The wages between $7,976 and $15,911 are taxed at 5.5%. The next tax brackets: $15,912 to $35,337 – 14%; $34,6211 to $94,735 – 30%; the wages higher than $94,735 are taxed at 41%.[12] There is a fixed 19% tax on capital gains from share sales and some bank interests; together with an additional 12.1% social tax, the capital gains tax jumps to 31.15%. As for the taxes paid by businesses, the standard "corporate tax rate" is 33.33% (though there are reduced rates of 16.5 and 15%); 3.3% of this is "social contributions." The French (including the businesses) also pay a huge 20.% VAT (value added tax) as a sales tax, with almost any purchase.[*13]

On paper, these taxes look prohibitive. However, almost all payroll deductions shown in the table are tax deductible! As a result, the actual tax paid is considerably less.

The French income tax system is quite sophisticated. Here is an interesting feature: A family with or without children after having deducted most social charges paid through payroll deductions, does not pay income tax in the bracket of the total (husband's plus wife's) wages. The family tax status is defined according to the so-called family quotient. Each adult has one share; the first two children –1/2, and the other children – 1 of a share each. The tax bracket is used for the income divided by the number of shares, and then the

---

[*] A reduced VAT rate is applied to "cultural products" such as books (in 2012 it isalso applied to e- books) as well as to food, drink, and public transportation. The "super reduced" VAT of 2.1% applies to "goods from chemists and some newspapers."

total tax is calculated according to the total family share number. This allows the family to come out of a higher tax bracket. In the U.S., our 1040 tax form also provides special tax allowances for dependents. However the French deductions are more radical. Even a family without children (the number of shares 2) pays taxes based on half of the combined husband and wife's income. A more impressive example: A typical middle class family with three children and an income of $80,000 have a family share of 4 (1+1+1/2x2 +1), and will pay tax from $20,000 in the tax bracket of 14% (rather than 30%).

Health care that is almost free covers those below 120% of the French Poverty Level (60% of median income), i.e., $14,818 (roughly 14% of the population); "almost free" because, as I mentioned, earnings above $7,975 (for a single) are taxable at 5.5%. A family will pay taxes based on its family quotient. Apart from paying taxes, those earning above $10,500 (singles), also have payroll deductions. Eyeglasses, hearing aids and dental prostheses are not free, although people pay discounted prices. For the very poor they are free but the waiting time is very long. Our Medicaid is more generous!

Most of the money deducted from paychecks is paid by the government directly into Social Security funds. All the funds are private, non-profit, and are operated by their Boards of Trustees. Most people are covered by three groups of funds, depending on their occupation: industrial and commerce employees and their families, agricultural workers, and the self-employed. There is also a variety of other funds: maternity leave allowance for pregnant women, family assistance, pensions (different funds for basic and supplementary pensions), and so forth. The government's role is only to supervise the funds' operation, insuring that the moneys received are used correctly. The government also supervises non-private hospitals.

As for the national doctor's fee schedule, it is not imposed by the government. The insurance funds negotiate these rates with leading physicians' associations and they are approved by a national convention.

As I mentioned, the French pay cash after every doctor visit or hospital stay and are later reimbursed from their Social Security funds. As we shall see, Social Security does not cover all health expenses. The rest (co-payment may be 10 to 40%) is picked up by supplemental private insurance: 80% of the population is enrolled in these supplemental programs.

Supplemental insurance (*Mutuelle*) is provided by private insurance companies. There are more than 300 for-profit and non-profit private insurance companies. They are independent and are more loosely regulated than insurance companies in the U.S. Typically, an enrollee may choose among three levels of coverage.[*] As a rule, enrollment is assisted by the employer. On average, employees pay about 2.5% of their wages for supplemental insurance.[†]

And now what the French buy for the money they pay. The list of how much is covered is impressive.[14,15]

- 70% of doctors' visits (generalists and specialists, including psychiatric care), plus €1 ($1.30) co-payment per visit (limited to $65 per year).
- 100% of doctors' visits for children age two and younger.
- 95-100% of prenatal care and childbirth.
- 65% of vaccinations (70% if the vaccination is given during regular doctor's appointments and 100% if the patient is considered to be "at risk" due to age or health problems).
- paramedical services (nurses, physical therapists, etc.): co-payment of $0.65 for each treatment, no more than $2.60 a day, with a limit of $65 per year.
- 70% of dental visits (this includes cavity treatments, tooth pulling, crowns, and bridges).
- 100% of orthodontic treatment for children younger than 16.
- 65% of eyeglass costs, limited to one pair per year.
- 65% of prescription drugs, depending on type (may be covered less) plus $0.65 for each prescription, with a copay limit of $65 per year.
- 60% of laboratory services, plus a flat rate co-payment of $1.30; 70% for x-rays.
- 100% of major health problems that last more than six months. HIV, Alzheimer's disease, Parkinson's disease, diabetes, hemophilia, cirrhosis of the liver, and others (from the list of 30 illnesses) are covered *completely*.
- 95% and 80% of major and minor surgeries respectively (70% of anesthesia treatments), plus a daily co-payment of $20 ($16 in a psychiatric unit) for in-hospital stay of up to 30 days.
- 100% of hospital charges for those who must be hospitalized longer

---

[*] The friends of mine – a typical middle-class family with three little children and both parents working– pay less than $150 monthly for an intermediate coverage. Insurance picks up everything unpaid by Social Security: 20% to 30% of the bills.
[†] The 2004 reform requires visits to specialists or specialized tests to be administered by primary care physicians. As I mentioned, there is resistance to this requirement, and there are ways to sidestep it. Then reimbursement is slashed. In principle, it could be covered by supplemental insurance. However, the government explicitly prohibits that!

than 30 days.

- 100% of hospital charges for women with birth complications, before and after delivery.

- 80% of home care; 100% for those with long-term illnesses.

- 100% of *cures thermales*, or spa hydrotherapy, for those with such debilitating long-term illnesses as neuropathy and inflammatory polyarthritis (this includes spa lodging up to $195 per night and a round-trip, second-class ticket on a SNCF train, as most French spas are on the coasts).

- transportation: 65% except for emergency cases; $2.60 per trip with a maximum of 2 trips a day and an annual ceiling of $65.

As one can see, the health care of adults, including prescription drugs, doctors' visits, and so on are on average reimbursed by 65-70%. As a poll has shown, in France only 7% of people with chronic conditions had to pay out-of-pocket costs higher than U.S. $1,000 (41% in the U.S.).[16]

The medical care of children, which begins with prenatal care, is reimbursed completely.

After having said so much about the French health care system, I have not yet discussed how a practicing physician works. As I mentioned earlier, more than 50 years ago, after fierce resistance, physicians agreed to accept the government's universal fee schedule. Today physicians are paid for their services by Social Security funds according to a standard tariff scheme. However, unlike American Medicare, some physicians are allowed to charge patients more,[*] but patients will still be reimbursed only at the standard rate.

An average French doctor earns about $55,000 per year, slightly more than one third of what an American doctor earns. Doctors' actual income is somewhat higher because the government pays two-thirds of their social security tax (this tax is typically 40% of income). To increase their income doctors may increase the number of patients they treat and administer more diagnostic tests. Physicians in France are no different than those in the U.S.

There are three reasons physicians agree to low incomes. They do not have the enormous debts that young American doctors have. Medical schools in France are free. Future doctors study four years less than American medical students.

---

[*] Some physicians are "more equal" than others. Depending on qualifications, a physician is either *secteur 1* or *secteur 2*. Tariffs in *secteur 1* are fixed (*tariff de convention*), whereas doctors in *secteur 2* can charge whatever fee they want (http://languedoc.angloinfo.com/countries/france/healthcare.asp). Over 25% of physicians do that, including those who have spent four years or more working in a hospital.

France

To enter a medical school a high school diploma is the only requirement[*] and malpractice insurance is not as destructive to doctors' practice as it often is in the U.S.

The national standard fees that doctors charge patients are as follows (fee/patient's co-pay),[†] and they are reimbursed at 70%: general consultation: $30/$9; specialist consultation: $33/$10.[17] There is also a $1.30 surcharge for every doctor visit.[‡]

The categories of specialists that a patient may see without a primary physician's referral include gynecologists, ophthalmologists, and psychiatrists (for those under age 26).

Apart from supervising the functioning of social security funds, the government's second function is to control the cost of drugs. Based on drug costs in neighboring countries, the Ministry of Health negotiates costs directly with pharmaceutical companies. The final decision on price is made by a board of doctors and experts that decides on the medical quality of the medicine worthy to be reimbursed. Most drugs are reimbursed, including homeopathy.

A few words about French hospitals.[18] Public and private hospitals and clinics exist side-by-side and compete for patients and prestige. Private hospitals are highly accessible and a patient has the right to choose a hospital of his/her liking.

The public hospitals charge standard fees whereas the private ones have their own charges, which are not always higher than those in public hospitals.

---

[*] To be accepted to a medical school in France, one does not need an undergraduate degree. What is required is a high school diploma with high marks in math, physics, chemistry, and biology. "High marks" means successfully passing matriculation exams (called *bacalaureat*). They include a written part and an oral part, each on several subjects, and last for up to six days. There are no multiple choice tests. Sixty-two percent of young people pass the exams. There are no admission tests for entrance to medical school. However, after the first year there is a selection test that allows only about 20% of the students to continue their medical studies (http://www.studentdoc.com/phpBB2/viewtopic.php?t=7981).
[†] The rates (and also whether the physician is *secteur 1* or *secteur 2*) must be clearly displayed in the physician's office.
[‡] A few years ago a €1 ($1.36) non-refundable surcharge on a medical visit was introduced in France, causing a minor mutiny. As my French friend wrote, "It was felt as a scandal by many people thinking about the poor old people who will have to pay the same tax as the rich. €1 is less than the price for a cup of coffee, but for the poor it is a loaf of bread." This is difficult for an American to understand. If it amounts to a loaf of bread, why not skip a doctor's visit if the complaint is just a headache?

Who Cares about Health Care?

Private hospitals accept "standard" fees but may charge more according to their tariffs; some private clinics may even charge less. Very few private hospitals operate completely outside the public sector; for those who do, supplemental insurance may cover the charges.

On the other hand, in public hospitals there may be consultants who have the right to charge patients at their own rates. Typically, the social security system reimburses hospital treatment at 80% of official rates, though there may be some extra costs that a patient or his/her supplemental insurance will have to pay.

Maternity care.[19] By law, pregnant women are eligible for 16 weeks of maternity leave: 6 weeks before and 10 weeks after the birth, and 26 weeks (8 + 18) for the third child;[*] fathers are also eligible for parental leave. While on leave the parent's job is preserved, and she/he receives an allowance.

> A pregnant woman is obliged to undergo seven antenatal examinations, which will be fully refunded. The first visit must take place before the end of the third month of pregnancy. After this examination, exams are monthly from the fourth month. Women not immune to toxoplasmosis will have their blood tested at a laboratory monthly. Generally, three sonograms will be conducted during a pregnancy.

> The postnatal period involves examinations for both the mother and infant. The baby is examined in the first week and then nine further times in the first year, three during the second, and two during each of the next years up to the sixth birthday. Of these exams, three contribute to a "certificate of good health" - the first week, ninth month and twenty-fourth month. The gynecologist examines both the mother and baby at eight weeks after delivery. Mothers are also prescribed and reimbursed for postnatal physical therapy. [19]

Almost all the expenses of pre- and postnatal care are covered by several social security funds; the extras may include, for example, giving birth in a private hospital or requesting a gynecologist to be present at the birth (unless it is medically necessary, in which case it is not an "extra").

---

[*] Maternity leave on the birth of twins: 34 weeks (12 before and 22 after delivery); for triplets: 46 weeks (24 + 22). If for some reason a woman wants to shorten her maternity leave, by law she *must* stop working for at least 8 weeks before and 6 weeks after delivery (http://vosdroits.service-public.fr/F2265.xhtml). In order to be completely covered, a pregnant woman has to register her pregnancy with a doctor. However, she does not have to inform her employer about her pregnancy until just before her maternity leave is to begin.

France

Although kindergartens are not a part of the health care system, I would like to say (as I did discussing Canada), just a few words about how they are organized in France.

Pre-school education in France (called *école maternelle* – "nursery school") is free and is run by the government (day-to-day operations are regulated by municipalities). It is not compulsory; however almost 100% of 3-5 year-old children attend (even 52% of 2-years-olds do).[*] Children attend nursery schools four days a week (with Wednesdays and weekends excluded), from three hours in the morning (8:30/9:00 to 11:30/12:00 AM), then, after lunch and a nap, three more hours (1:30/2:00 to 4:00/4:30, PM). The French believe that pre-school education plays an important role in their children's lives and take it seriously.

> Nursery school is designed to introduce children to the social environment of school and to develop the basic coordination skills. The main aim of nursery schooling is oral expression and communication. Self-awareness is encouraged as well as group activities. These include arts and crafts, music, and games. During the final years of nursery school, the rudiments of reading, writing, and arithmetic are taught in preparation for Primary school.

> For parents not used to the nursery school system, sending a child to school at three years old may seem premature. However, the French nursery system is excellent, and not only a way to help children socialize but to make long-lasting friends. A child who enters the French system at Primary school level may well find it much harder not only to succeed but to integrate.[20]

Now turning to the elderly. France's social security system provides universal long-term care (LTC) care insurance. Like the rest of its health care, this insurance is based on payroll deductions and taxes and the benefits are closely tied to income.[21]

Only 30% of LTC is covered by public funds. People over age 65 who need long-term care receive a subsidy regardless of their financial situation. However, co-payment can reach 80% of the cost; only low-income people are exempted from it.

---

[*] My French friends recently (2013) attempted to enroll their two years old son to *école maternelle,* but were refused acceptance. The school was full above its capacity: in my friends' Paris suburb middle class families have 4-5 children. However, a three year old may not be turned down by the school. So, my friends will have to wait…

To supplement their public benefits, one-quarter of the elderly have purchased private LTC insurance. This issue is being actively discussed in the media, and the market for private LTH care insurance is booming in France, increasing by 15% a year, in spite of the fact that no tax incentives are used to encourage purchasing private insurance. Most policies provide a fixed allowance with monthly cash payments regardless of whether the money will be spent for home or for nursing home care.[22]

Nursing home costs vary from $80 to $220 a day, or $29,000 to $81,000 per year. This is at least 1.5-2 times less expensive than in the U.S.

To find a nursing home in a desired location and of appropriate quality is not easy, though there are also a variety of assisted living complexes, exactly like in the U.S. Typically, they are blocks of one- or two-room apartments. For example, in Paris and the Paris region there are 46 residential homes that accommodate about 3000 elderly who are self-sufficient and can live independently.

How is a medical emergency handled in France?

> Emergency medical services in France are provided by a mix of organizations under public health control, with the lead taken by a central control function called SAMU, which stands for "Service d'Aide Médicale Urgente" or urgent medical aid service. This central hub is supported by resources including first response vehicles or ambulances provided by the fire service and physician-led ambulance provision from SMUR (Service Mobile d'Urgence et Reanimation - literally translated as mobile emergency and resuscitation service) which are "mobile intensive care units" (MICU) that have one or more physicians on board.[23]

If the case is not serious, an emergency vehicle affiliated with a fire station may be sent. It will administer first aid and bring the patient to a hospital. In more serious cases a SAMU vehicle will be sent. The decision of what kind of vehicle to send and how it should be manned will be made by a doctor who answers the French equivalent of a 911 call. SAMU stays with the patient longer than paramedics do because the doctor in charge begins treatment before the patient has been brought to the most appropriate hospital and during the ride.* All the emergency expenses are paid from social security

---

* After the tragic car accident in a Paris tunnel that resulted in Princess Diana's death, it took two hours before she was brought to a hospital. The media then accused the attending doctors of being too slow administering first aid, rather than rushing Diana to a hospital right away. Possibly those accusations were unfounded.

funds.

Throughout this chapter, I have been comparing some aspects of French and American health care systems.

Like Canada, France has a higher life expectancy, lower child mortality, and lower death rates from heart disease, stroke, and respiratory disease than other countries. Although France has more hospital beds and doctors per capita than the U.S., the main difference in delivering treatment, like in Canada, comes from the disparity of health care between Caucasians and minority populations in America. In Canada and France everybody is equally covered by health care services (for children and pregnant women, some services are even mandatory, under the threat of losing coverage), whereas in the U.S. it is a money matter.

The huge difference in deaths from diabetes is an exception: it is a consequence of the obesity epidemic in the U.S.

The French, like the Canadians, visit doctors more often than Americans: an obvious manifestation of moral hazard: if one knows that a doctor is easily available, one schedules an appointment. In France, however, the moral hazard is somewhat eased by the necessity to pay cash after each doctor visit: Though people know that they are covered and will be reimbursed, nobody wants to pay money upfront!

An important feature of the French health-care system is the *Carte Vitale* – a plastic card that is the main identification for all medical purposes. The card contains all the administrative information necessary for the monetary transactions that have to do with the care: [24]

-Social Security number
-Details of the health insurance plan
-Details of the relevant health insurance office (address, phone number, etc.)
-Full name and date of birth of the cardholder and dependents
-Details of any exemption or reduction that apples to payments or entitlement to supplementary universal coverage.
-The *Carte Vitale* does not include personal medical information. Upon arriving at an appointment, the patient produces the card and the doctor slides it through the computer. After the appointment, the doctor enters the code of the treatment on the card. This information will be automatically sent to the appropriate health fund. The patient's reimbursement is sent to the patient's bank accounts. The fee for supplemental insurance (if any) will be taken from the patient's account. No bills, no hassle! Millions of dollars in savings!

To summarize: the French health care system is quite efficient, both in quality of care and distribution of funds,[*] but it is expensive. And yet the French love it! Some 65% of French citizens are satisfied with their system, whereas in the U.S. only 40% are satisfied. The French are proud of their health care system. Moreover, as a 2005 survey shows, "three best symbols of the French nation are the flag, the health and the *Marseillaise*" (quoted in[1]).

I would like to end this chapter with the following quote:

> Several salient features of the French health care system – the dominance of office-based private practice (la médecine libérale) for ambulatory care, the mix of public and private hospitals, the widespread use of cost sharing, the predominant practice of direct payment from patient to doctor, and the reliance upon financing derived from payroll taxes – resemble elements of the U.S. health system. These points of convergence make French national health insurance especially relevant to Americans interested in learning from abroad. This is all the more true given the current prospects for health care reform and the interest in proposals for employer-financed national health insurance.[25]

Germany

The Federal Republic of Germany (*Bundesrepublik Deutschland*) is a federation of sixteen states ("lands"). Among the members of the European Union, it is the most populous nation (81.3 million) with the strongest economy.

The history of Germany in the 20th century is turbulent and tragic. As I already mentioned, Otto von Bismarck united numerous German states into the German Empire in 1871. The Empire was a militaristic, aggressive state that was instrumental in unleashing World War I.

The war was terrible and irrational. The machine gun, an efficient killing device, was an innovation of that war. Germany was the first in the history of humankind to use poison gas (the term weapons of mass destruction, WMD, did not yet exist).

After four bloody years (1914-1918), leaving 10 million dead, the Allied

---

[*] It has a very low administrative cost: 5% of the total expenditure as compared with 14% in the U.S. (http:// www.brookings.edu/articles/2002/07france_dutton.aspx).

Powers: Britain, France and the U.S. won; the third partner, Russia, had just succumbed to a Communist revolution. The Central Powers: Germany and its allies, the Austro-Hungarian and Ottoman empires were crushed. The Treaty of Versailles established peace in Europe. However, the heavy reparations imposed on Germany (that it was virtually unable to pay) are believed to have paved the way for the Nazis.

The so-called Weimar Republic, proclaimed in 1918, had been suffocating for a decade under enormous inflation and later the Great Depression. In 1933 the Nazis came to power and inflamed the world with World War II.

WWII, unparalleled in the world's history in its victims – both human and material – has changed the world forever. The Holocaust has proved that millions of people can be easily and ruthlessly murdered to glorify an idea. The nuclear weapon emerged. People lost their faith in humanity.

When WWII was over, Germany was lying in shambles. Soon after the war's end the Cold War began. Within a decade Germany was split into the Federal Republic of Germany which, thanks to the Marshall Plan, was rebuilt into a flourishing democratic state, and the German Democratic Republic, a Soviet satellite, which was allowed to stagnate for another 45 years until in 1990, after the fall of Communism, it was reunited with the Federal Republic.

This short review of German history is meant to emphasize the unbelievable contrast: During the 130 years of that dramatic history, Germany had fundamentally the same health care system! Von Bismarck's 1883 health care legislation was the foundation of a health care model (which now bears his name) that was later adopted by many European states. Its principles stayed unchanged during the turmoil's of history.

Before turning to today's Germany, I would like to say a few words about health care in Nazi Germany.[1]

During the 30s, the so-called Social Darwinism, the "theory" that appeared a decade earlier before the Nazis came to power, became popular, making an impact on the Nazi health care system. Social Darwinism fitted the Nazi ideology well. Its bottom line was that the physically and mentally inferior, homosexuals, and the handicapped were "unworthy of living" and had to be eliminated. As for the "racially inferior," they simply had to be liquidated en masse. The multi-million people genocide, including the Holocaust, the murder of six million Jews, was the ultimate realization of the Nazis' ideology.

Most Germans supported the Nazi regime and were even patriotic. People of the medical profession and scientists in general were no exception. Close to half of the nation's medical doctors and the majority of biologists were members of the Nazi party.

The Nazis heavily supported medical research. The Germans were the first to firmly establish that smoking causes lung cancer (that information was deliberately hidden after the end of WWII by the victors, for the benefit of tobacco companies), and that asbestos was harmful. The entire Nazi health care system was directed at preserving the good health of the "nation." Special attention was paid to children's and women's health, hygiene, healthy work conditions, etc. Dr. Robert N. Proctor writes: [2]

> There is nothing wrong with physicians working to preserve the health of a larger community; that, after all, is the essence of responsible public health. What differentiated National Socialist public health from genuine public health in a reasonably civilized society was the exclusive nature of what the Nazis considered "the community." Nazi values excluded Jews and others deemed racially or genetically unfit from the völkisch community.

Both medical research and regular health care in Nazi Germany had an ideological underpinning: to make the Aryan Third Reich healthy, not only freeing it from sicknesses, but also eliminating what were considered subhuman contaminating elements.

Most doctors worked at clinics and hospitals. Among them, thousands were secretly experimenting on inmates in prisons and concentration and death camps. An army of anthropologists were studying "low race" physical features in people (like the shape of the head) and identifying those "unworthy of living."

One of the first Nazi laws, passed in July 1933, was the "Law for the Prevention of Progeny of Hereditary Disease." It was the first law of this kind. Others followed. A "Genetic Health Court" was established which, by decisions of judges and doctors in closed sessions lasting just a few minutes, sentenced the "genetically inferior" to sterilization or euthanasia. Close to half a million people were forcibly sterilized. Thousands of handicapped children were murdered at birth.

Of course, there were physicians who refused to collaborate with the regime, but they were a silent minority.

Unfortunately, I was unable to find any information about how the Nazi health system worked. Most probably, in the spirit of Bismarck, it was a one-payer system, where the bills were paid directly by the government and patients never saw them. Non-Aryan patients were probably refused treatment. Did a patient had to wait for a long time before being admitted by a doctor or to a hospital? Most probably. The system was efficient, as efficient as their mass murder machine. And probably, most Germans, peacefully awaiting doctors' appointments in clinics, or being treated in hospitals or nursing homes, did not even know about the Nazis' crimes.[*]

Since the end of WWII, Germany's Bismarck–model-based health care has been a dynamic system, endlessly changing through both minor and serious reforms. In the past 20 years, health care reforms were enacted at least six times: about every three years. The most recent reform was passed by the Reichstag in November 2010.

The main goal of Bismarck's reform (in his own words, as I quoted in the Introduction) was protection of the employee. Therefore, to this day, the so-called *statutory social security system* guaranteeing the employee's well being still exists in Germany. The following pillars are the foundation of the system: health insurance, unemployment insurance, old-age pensions, long-term care insurance, and accident insurance.

The German system is quite expensive. Judging by the GDP chunk spent on health care (11.3%), it is the fourth after the U.S.'s 17.6% (and follows 11.6% of France). As of 2013, Germany had an €13 ($17)[†] billion deficit; therefore slashing health-care expenditure has been the main goal of German governments for years.

Today, the German health-care package covers:[3] preventive services, both inpatient and outpatient care in hospitals, outpatient physician services, mental health care, dental services, prescription drugs, necessary medical supplies, rehabilitation services, and maternity and sick leave payments. Since 1995 long-term care has also been covered.

Health care in Germany is universal and multi-payer: all German citizens and residents (as well as migrant workers) must enroll in either the public or a private plan. It is simply illegal to be uninsured. (See an informative "Questions and Answers" site.[4])

---

[*] I have promised to be non-partisan. However, and I hope my readers will agree with me, comparison of Obama's health care reform with racially motivated medicine in Nazi Germany by numerous bloggers and prominent right-wing politicians is not just ridiculous: it is immoral. I completely agree with the following quote from a comment by Dr. Arthur Caplan, director of the Center for Bioethics at the University of Pennsylvania (http://www.msnbc.msn.com/id/32372258/ns/health-health care/): "Their flagrant, deliberate and invidious distortion of what happened to medicine in Nazi Germany must not be allowed to stand. Not just because health reform is too important an issue but also because the truth is too important to let ignoramuses destroy it."

[†] I will be converting Euros into dollars (€1=$1.36).

Who Cares about Health Care?

The backbone of German public health care is a conglomerate of about 140 *Krankenkassen*, "sickness funds" (SFs): non-profit funds providing necessary services. They are completely self-sufficient and pay for medical services directly to providers. The SFs are government controlled but not a part of government bureaucracy. In this respect, today's German health care is not a single-payer one: it is the SF that pays one's bills, rather than the government.

If a German earns below $68,380 (2013)[3], enrollment in SFs is mandatory. If one's gross income exceeds $68,380 one may opt out of the public option and purchase instead private (for-profit) health insurance. Some 7% of Germans choose to rely on private insurance. If the insurance company is German (and about 50 such companies are available), and can produce a special government certificate, then the insured is eligible for a subsidy from his/her employer of the same amount as if the employee had chosen public rather than private insurance. Moreover, the insurance company has to put 10% of one's premiums aside as a contribution to a retirement plan.

All who are employed by a German company and wish to stay in public system may enroll in an SF. If one does, the medical expenses are split almost 50-50 between the employer and the employee (in Bismarck's original model it was 1/3 - 2/3). Up to a total annual income of $61,900 or $5,160 per month, an employee pays a standardized premium (independent of the SF one is enrolled in) through payroll deductions: 8.3% of one's gross salary; 7.3% is paid by the employer, with the total of 15.5%.* However, if one earns more than the above threshold, one's deduction is still based on a $5,160 monthly salary (of which 8.3% deduction is $428).

Since 2009 private insurance companies were not allowed to arbitrarily charge the insured. A mandatory government monthly premium tariff was established for the private companies. This tariff completely disregards age, gender, and, what is most important, health status (the infamous "pre-existing conditions") – exactly as in public health insurance. On top of that the insurance companies are not allowed to charge the insured more than $650 per month. (" . . . you can bet whatever is dear to you that the average premium will be like $649.99 eventually as a result."[5])

As one can see, affluent people could, in principle stay with SFs: it would not be more expensive than for people of moderate income. The main reason for switching to a private health plan is to expand the benefits. The public option does not cover a private doctor/surgeon or a private room in a hospital nor does it cover alternative/homeopathic medical care or eyeglasses for adults. Dental

---

* Wage limits and rates of contributions are annually set by the German parliament (Bundestag).

care is covered from 20 to 70%, although implants are not covered. Services outside Europe are not covered either. The SF will not pay if one needs to consult a distinguished medical figure such as a hospital department head. One can improve one's benefits by purchasing a supplemental private insurance without leaving the public domain. Some 9% of Germans do that.

On the other hand, the public option automatically covers spouses, children and elderly parents, whereas private insurance requires separate policies for each family member.

There is a special category of people who are also eligible for private health insurance. These are the self-employed, people in the artistic professions, and civil service workers. However, health care options for the self-employed and regular employees differ: the self-employed must take care for their own health-care and old-age survival as they are not covered by any public social security. They also do not have unemployment benefits. This is the legacy of Bismarck's nineteenth-century social security system.[6]

Nevertheless, since 2009, self-employed workers are also required to have insurance. Like in the U.S., they have to pay their social security dues – the whole 15.5% – from their pockets.[*] The number of self-employed people in Germany rises from year to year, women contributing considerably to the numbers.

Let me return to private insurance. Someone who decides to opt out of the public system has to think twice: having left for private insurance, one is not allowed to return to the public option even if one's income drops below the $68,380 threshold. Against the background of the generally humane German health care system this regulation seems strange: it is obviously mistreating the self-employed.[†]

---

[*] The corresponding rules are extremely complex: websites advising expatriates wishing to return to Germany suggest discussing the self-employment issue with competent experts. Low-income self-employed have government subsidies. There is an interesting way of dealing with the unemployed who are eligible for a government start-up grant (so-called bridge money), which covers both modest subsistence and a monthly allowance of $780, $480, and $310 respectively for the first, second and third year.

[†] A telling example comes to mind. Suppose a person has successfully worked for a high-tech company, and achieved a pretty high salary. The person has ideas that could result in a successful business and decides to start his/her own company. The person's official employment category immediately changes from "employee" to "self-employed" (while still on one's own), and then to "employer." Suppose the company is not successful (in the U.S. some 80% of start-up companies go broke). Now the person is out in the cold: the private policy is expensive and now has to be

Who Cares about Health Care?

A medical doctor who is not employed by a hospital often belongs to either the "self-employed" category (having an office in his/her apartment with a brass plate on the wall reading, for example, Herr/Frau **Dr. Schmidt, neurologist) or the "employer" category if he/she has small clinic with other doctors, nurses and other ancillary personnel. However,** among 134,000 outpatient practices, doctors working solo prevail.

Germany has almost 1.5 times more practicing physicians than the U.S. (3.8 vs. 2.5 per 1000 population, in 2011). Therefore there is practically no waiting if one needs to see a specialist. Wait time for an appointment is actually less than that in the U.S.

Often, small private clinics or single doctors join forces in negotiation with SFs, but they typically do not coordinate their patient treatment. The competition among doctors is fierce! Doctors bill patients according to standard government reimbursement rates –"tariffs" – on every possible service. Well, they don't bill patients literally: patients never see their bills. For them visit to a doctor is "free." Doctors send the bills to the corresponding SFs and are reimbursed accordingly.

German hospitals comprise a vast and diverse realm. To begin with, they are under diverse ownership: private and government, non-profit and for-profit: About 54% of hospitals are in the public sector, about 38% are private, non-profit, and some 8% are private, for-profit institutions. When it comes to hospital services, queues are unheard of. There is, however a discrimination of "public" patients with respect of those insured privately: hospitals are interested in "live" money; therefore a private patient goes first.

As in the case of outpatient services (and typically hospitals do not provide them) hospital patients do not see their bills. Hospitals are also reimbursed by SFs according to the number of days a patient stays, rather than services rendered. On average, a patient stays in a German hospital for 9.5 days: twice as long as in the U.S. Private insurance bills, however, may be enormous.

Standard hospitals have two-bed rooms, though some may have larger wards. A patient can request a single room with a copayment that can even be more than $100.

The government does not micromanage doctors and hospitals. The global budget and the list of procedures eligible for coverage are set and approved by the National Association of Sickness Funds and the National Association of Physicians. However, the reimbursement rates are regulated by the

---

paid from a lower income, until he/she finds a new job and becomes an "employee" again.

government.[*]

Actually, the government tariffs fix only *baseline* reimbursement rates. These rates are considerably higher for serious illnesses like cancer, AIDS, or others – out of the list of 80 high-cost illnesses.

Having collected payroll deductions from all participating in the public option, the government transfers the money to corresponding SFs. Some SFs are small, having just a few thousand enrollees; in a few large SFs millions are enrolled. Thus, every SF accumulates a pool of money which, in principle, should be enough to cover its enrollees: that is, to pay the bills from their service providers. However, because the reimbursement rates are just average numbers, in some situations a doctor's bill for a procedure will exceed the tariff. If it is justified, the SF must pay. As a result, there may be a situation where the SF's budget is not enough to pay all the bills. A simple example is a flu epidemic. The government may or may not decide to bail out such an SF. Therefore it is necessary for each SF to keep its budget intact. This results in fierce competition among SFs for their enrollees, who inevitably feel when their SF is in the cold (i.e., doctors complain that payments for their services have been delayed) and may switch to another SF. Although the SFs are non-profit funds, they have to pay their overhead expenses and therefore must be efficient. An example: SFs have to pay for their enrollees' prescription drugs. By directly negotiating with pharmaceutical companies, SFs can achieve drug prices that are below the reference prices set by the government, thus making their individual budgets more stable. Some SFs do become bankrupt.

Unlike in Canada, France, and American HMOs, in Germany one does not need an internist's referral to see a specialist. The Germans are not restricted in their right to choose any doctor. And they do use that right to spur doctors' competition.

> Consumers can and do penalize bad service. Our recent study of German consumers commonly produced reactions like this: "I saw a long queue, so hopped on the subway and went to a different practice"; "she was rather ill-tempered so I never went back"; "the facilities were drab, so I went to a different one next to my office"; "I felt rushed at his practice so didn't go back".[7]

---

[*] By law, a fee may be higher, by up to a factor of 3.5. In that case, a doctor must justify the increase, for example by insisting that the procedure was complicated and time consuming. A doctor can also negotiate a definite price increase with a patient in advance. (http://www.justlanded.com/english/Germany/Articles/Health/Hospital-and-doctor-s-bills). However, for the patient the price for treatment is irrelevant because the bills are paid directly by SFs anyway. __

Who Cares about Health Care?

Since 2004, in order to contain costs, the Germans have to pay a copayment of $6.50 to $13 for prescription drugs (depending on the size of the drug package), $13 for each hospital stay, and $13 each quarter when visiting a doctor (either an internist or a specialist).

This $13 is paid to the first doctor seen in the quarter. If a consultation with another doctor is necessary, one has to produce a referral from the first doctor. Otherwise, another $13 copayment must be paid. Without additional copayments one may have to pay $52 in one year. However the maximum personal expenditure for different copayments (e.g., for prescription drugs or staying in hospital) is capped to 2% of one's gross income. Patients with chronic illnesses do not have to pay more than 1%.[8] Vaccination and doctor visits for low-income patients and children younger than 18 are exempt from copayment. If one uses emergency services in the same quarter, one has to pay $13 again.

Like everywhere in Europe, a medical doctor does not expect to earn much money. Upon beginning his/her practice, a physician in Germany does not have any tuition debts. As in France, medical school education is free.[*]

On average, a German doctor makes about 1/3 of what an American doctor makes. In 2005 German doctors went on strike. However, with the current financial situation (a huge deficit) they cannot hope for a significant increase in earnings.[†]

Malpractice insurance is not as troublesome as in the U.S. Partly, because German doctors do not purchase malpractice insurance from for-profit insurance companies, but rather from medical protective associations, which is much cheaper. There are also almost no frivolous lawsuits: contingency fees ("pay if won") are prohibited and the plaintiff pays trial expenses if the case is lost.

---

[*] Like in France, to be eligible to apply to a medical school, one has to achieve high marks on the so-called *Abiture* – high school matriculation exams. Admission is administered jointly by the university and a centralized government organization. In the first two years of medical school, the so-called pre-clinical classes, students study the basic disciplines of physics, chemistry, biology, anatomy, physiology, biochemistry, etc. Those who pass a federal national medical exam continue their study for another four years (including clinical specialization). After the last, so-called practical year and the final federal exam, students receive a license and the title of M.D. In order to be allowed to have an independent practice, a physician has to pass residency in a chosen specialization field for three to six years. (http://en.wikipedia.org/wiki/Medical_school#Germany).

[†] In such a situation brain drain among doctors is inevitable. It has an interesting dynamic: German doctors try to find jobs in France and Switzerland, whereas Eastern European doctors migrate to Germany.

A word on maternity benefits.[9] The population level cannot be maintained if the fertility rate is lower than 2.1 per woman. However, Germany has an alarmingly low fertility rate of 1.39 (as of 2011[*10]). This is a serious issue. The situation is becoming more alarming because the Muslim emigrants have a much higher fertility rate that significantly shifts the ethnic equilibrium.

The law guarantees maternity leave of 12 weeks: 6 weeks before and 6 weeks after the birth. In case of multiple births or danger to the life of mother and/or child, the leave can be extended.

Actually, the leave is 12 months if only the mother takes it. The total parental leave is 14 months and it can be shared by both parents. If only the mother takes the leave, she is entitled to full income if she worked for at least 12 months before her pregnancy. If the father takes the leave (after the child is born), his employer reimburses 67% of his salary (or 65% for a salary above a certain threshold), but not more than $2,340 per month (on average fathers get $1,520 monthly). The parent may extend his/her leave without pay for up to three years; during this time the parent cannot be fired, and his/her position is saved.

Parental benefits are not restricted to the period of a child's birth. All children under the age of 18 receive an allowance, irrespective of their parents' income. In 2009, the monthly allowance was $215 for each of the first two children, $220 for the third child, and $255 for each subsequent child.

Parental benefits in Germany are quite generous but it does not stimulate fertility. A serious social issue is that many Germans believe that a woman should stay home before children reach school age, rather than advance her own career. And this is in spite of the fact that the percentage of families with both parents working is growing, and such families cannot afford many children.

Although close to 90 percent of children three to five years old are eligible for public or subsidized kindergartens, only 1/3 of them use child-care full time. Most pre–schools work only half-day, or children have to go home for lunch during a two-hour midday break; the school vacations are usually longer than work vacations, sometimes the vacation times do not coincide, and to find child–care during a work vacation is extremely difficult.[11] In short: the German pre-school child–care system is not organized such as to help working mothers, at a deep contrast with the French system.

---

[*] Such a low fertility rate is not typical of European countries. Some countries have a rate approaching the critical one (2011): Iceland – 2.02; Ireland – 2.05; France – 2.03; Norway – 1.88; Great Britain– 1.94; Sweden – 1.90; Finland –1.83, and Denmark–1.75.

Now to discuss long-term health care (LTC): [12] What the Germans have achieved after 1995 when long-term health care became mandatory is fantastic.

Long-term health care is a part of the social security package, but it is separate from regular health-care and unemployment insurance. It is also financed through payroll: from 2.02% to 2.3% of the monthly gross income (but not more than $135/month) is deducted, split equally between the employee and employer.

"Home care over facility-based care" is the main principle around which the whole, rather complex LTC care system revolves. To begin with, those eligible (over 65 years old) are subdivided into three levels, depending on the severity of their condition and their ability to fulfill daily living activities. This allows direct financing (numbers for 2010: 1st–3rd level/month): cash payable directly to the insured: $290 – $890; payments for nursing or other "in-kind" services – $570–$1,960.[13]

Although nursing homes are much less expensive than in the U.S., funds supplied by the public system are not sufficient to cover their expenses. The total cost of staying in a nursing home, depending on the assigned patient's level, varies from $2,950 to $4,270 /month ($95 – $140 /day), of which roughly 45% is paid by insurance. The rest is the patient's copayment: $1,620 to $2,310.[12,18] As we can see, it is significant.

Long-term health care is administered through SFs, which are different from those administering regular health care. However, there is no competition among them because the prices have been fixed by the government. Around 90% of Germans are enrolled in a public LTH care system whereas some 10% prefer a private one; enrollment in either of the systems is mandatory. In 2008 Germany spent on LTH 1.3% (0.9% from public sector expenses) of its GDP.

Another benefit that is worth mentioning is sick leave, which looks like an entitlement but is not, for it is paid for by employees through payroll deductions. The employer is responsible for paying the worker's full salary for up to six weeks; thereafter the *Krankenkasse* (SF) pays 70% of gross earnings (up to a maximum of 90% of net earnings). Benefits are paid for up to 78 weeks in a three-year period for the same illness. To the mother of a sick child benefit is paid for up to 10 working days per child, but up to 25 days per calendar year, even if more than one child was sick. In household with single parent, the benefit times are doubled respectively to 20 and 50 days.[14]

The sick unemployed are eligible for the same benefits as part of unemployment insurance. It is mandatory and is paid by the employee through payroll deduction. The amount is 6.5% of gross monthly earnings split equally with the employer.[15]

Emergency services.[16] Studying France, and now Germany, I was looking for information on emergency rooms but was unable to find it. As I mentioned, the French emergency service is different from what we have in America: an emergency phone call is answered by a doctor and doctors often man ambulances (remember the controversy over Princess Diana's death?).

Now I understand what the problem is: France and Germany typically *do not have emergency rooms at all!*[17] The main difference between the Franco-German emergency system and ours is that in America *the patient is brought to the doctor*, whereas in France and Germany *the doctor is brought to the patient*. In non–-life-threatening situations, rather than calling an ambulance, one calls his/her internist, who will visit the patient at home (24-7); very infrequently do such patients seek out emergency departments. In life-threatening situations, the first to arrive on the scene are paramedics. They may do defibrillation, administer life-saving drugs, and take other urgent measures until an MD arrives with a more sophisticated ambulance. The treatment begins in the ambulance, and, if necessary, the patient is brought directly to a hospital, in most cases already diagnosed, to the appropriate *emergency department*. In 80% of calls, an emergency vehicle arrives within 10 minutes, and in 95% of cases within 15 minutes.

Unlike the U.S. where the doctor in the emergency room is a regular MD (or a resident), the emergency doctors in Germany have special training: they are *emergency MDs*.

Such a system, which has existed for many years, began gradually giving way to a unified emergency treatment in hospitals, the way it is in the U.S. Most European countries now have U.S.-type emergency services.

Before I end my tour of German health care, just a few more pieces of information.

•Like in France, every German carries a Health-Care Card. It contains the person's name in electronic form as well as the person's picture, and identifies the SF in which the patient is enrolled. Like in France, billing and reimbursement are paperless. The German card is a version of the European E111 health insurance card.

• Germany has four times fewer MRI units and two times fewer CT scanners per capita than the U.S. Most probably, it is (like in Canada) because medical for-profit organizations are not as purchase-capable as in the U.S. Nevertheless, unlike Canada, in Germany there are no queues for diagnostic tests such as MRI or CT-scan.

Statistics show that in Germany life expectancy is higher and child mortality is

---

lower than in the U.S. I have already discussed these issues with respect to Canada. The higher child mortality rate in the U.S. is a consequence of American doctors' devotion to saving the lives of children who would not survive in other countries. The lower life expectancy in the U.S. reflects high level of violent deaths and accidents, as well as the inaccessibility of treatment for a large percentage of the population rather than the quality of care. • And just a short note on what the German doctors treat most often. The top diagnoses for males are heart disease, alcohol-related issues, and hernias; for females, the top diagnoses concern pregnancies, breast cancer, and heart disease.

I believe I have covered most of the important aspects of the German health-care system. The most fundamental principle, "employee über alles," that was laid as a foundation of German health care by Bismarck, is still the leading rule today. Actually, the employer is the true coordinator of health care, rather than just someone who shares expenses. The entire German system today is the manifestation of "practical Christianity," as envisioned by Bismarck and is seen by the Germans today.

Probably the most important issue that is already crying for reform in the U.S. is LTC. In 2011 German LTC, which is much better than ours, was the subject of discussions on the level of OECD (The Organization for Economic Cooperation and Development). There, AARP Board Chair Phil Zarlengo gave a keynote address entitled *Life After the Baby Boomers*.[1] The gist of his presentation was that, in the season of health-care reforms, Americans have much to learn from Germans [2].

If we could learn at least that one lesson, it would be a blessing for millions of American elderly.

Japan

Japan (Nippon-koku in Japanese) is located in the Pacific Ocean on an archipelago of 6,852 islands. With a population over 127 million, it is one of the most populated nations in the world and is the third largest economic power.

Japan is a constitutional monarchy. The power of Emperor Akihito, like the power of Queen Elizabeth of England, is limited. The constitution defines the Emperor as "the symbol of the state and the unity of the people."

—

Legislative power belongs to the *diet*, a parliament composed of the House of Representatives (480 members elected for four years) and the House of Councilors (252 members elected for six years). Executive power is exercised by a cabinet appointed and headed by the prime minister, who is elected by the *diet*. The official currency of Japan is the *yen* (¥).[*]

Even as recently as 150 years ago, the Emperor was still adored as a god, and was called and believed to be "the son of Heaven." However, for 800 years before the middle of the 19th century the emperor's power was quite limited, although he was the head of a sophisticated feudal hierarchy based on military clans of the samurai. The true power was in hands of shoguns – military warlords. For many centuries Japan existed in complete isolation from Europe, although the influence of China was significant. Penetration of Europeans from Portugal and England began only in the 16th –17th centuries.

Beginning with the year 1854, when an American flotilla of steam-powered military ships under the command of Commodore Matthew Perry sailed into Tokyo Bay, Japan's seclusion was over. As a result of economic, political, and cultural reforms, Japan became a unified and centralized nation. The 91-year period that lasted until Japan's defeat in WWII was one of economic development and growth against a background of absolutism and militarism – the legacy of centuries of military rule and expansionism.

The Japanese health care system was born in 1927: the *Employee Health Insurance Plan*. It covered only private sector employees and the insurance was only partial: dependents were not covered and benefits did not extend beyond 180 days.

At that time Japan was facing the challenge of fighting epidemics, with tuberculosis the most dangerous among them. In 1938 the Ministry of Health care was formed that eventually became a single authority controlling public health. By 1943, over 95% of municipalities were covered by national health insurance.[3]

In 1937 Japan invaded China and was waging war until it was crushed in 1945. During the war the Kenpei-Kenmin (Healthy Soldier, Healthy People) policy was implemented which, among other things, was focused on the health of mothers, as in Nazi Germany. In spite of shortages, pregnant women received rations of food and medical supplies.

On December 7, 1941, Japan attacked Pearl Harbor. America was awakened

---

[*] As of May 2014, ¥1= $0.216. As in the previous chapters, I will be giving financial information in U.S. dollars.

from its isolationism. After almost four years of bloody war, culminated by the American nuclear attack on Hiroshima and Nagasaki, Japan surrendered.[*]

The post-war history of Japan is just short of being a miracle, and is the triumph of the American Administration. By the Administration's incessant work on rebuilding the nation, Japan has turned from a totalitarian, militaristic and bloodthirsty aggressor into a flourishing democracy with a powerful economic and well-functioning health care system.[†] Today Japan also has the highest literacy rate in the world, and one of the lowest poverty rates.[4]

After the war was over, the social security and health-care systems were rebuilt. Health insurance at that time was based on individual insurance policies. In 1952, in order to subsidize government-controlled health insurance, the central government, for the first time, set aside one billion yen.[5] In 1961 the Universal Health Insurance law was passed. By 1984 the Japanese health care system became well functioning. Here are the most important highlights of its evolution:

1961: Universal coverage.
1962: Establishment of the Social Insurance Agency.
1972: Free medical care for the elderly.
1973: Revision of the Health Insurance Law (so-called First Year of Welfare State).
– Improvement of benefit level for families of the insured from 50% to 70%.
– Introduction of the upper ceiling for patients' cost sharing.
– National subsidy of 10% of health expenditure for government-managed health insurance.
1982: Law of Health and Medical Services for the Elderly (implementation: 1983).

---

[*] The militaristic propaganda in Japan during the war resulted in the unheard-of atrocities perpetrated on war prisoners. Twenty-five percent of American prisoners died, some of them cruelly executed (even in Nazi POW camps only 1% of Americans died, though the Nazis are infamous for their brutal genocidal policies). The propaganda turned the Japanese into fanatical automatons. Not only were the thousands of kamikaze willingly dying, causing severe losses among Americans; even civilians were sometimes willing to commit suicide rather than meet "bloodthirsty" American soldiers. And on the day Japan's surrender was announced, thousands of officers committed *hara-kiri* – traditional samurai suicide by disembowelment. Mass harakiri was performed on the square before the Emperor's palace: human intestines were everywhere.
[†] According to the recent Bloomberg ratings Japan is No. 3 in health care efficiency, and No 5 among the healthiest nations. (http://www.bloomberg.com/ visual-data/best-and-worst/most-efficient-health-care-countries;
http://images.businessweek.com/bloomberg/pdfs/worlds_healthiest_countries_V2.pdf).

1984: Revision of the Health Insurance Law.
– 10% cost sharing by the insured.
– Relaxation of regulations on high technology health care.
– Introduction of the health care program for retired persons.[3]

The beginning of the post-war health care system (1952) coincided with the withdrawal of the American Administration. It is interesting that, in spite of the decisive influence of the Administration on virtually every sphere of Japanese life, Japan refused to follow the American model of health care, instead joining Europe in developing "health-care-for-all."   Japan closely follows the "practical Christianity" Bismarck model. Was it because the nation that had suffered so much truly needed humane health care?

Today, "Japan has a system that costs half as much and often achieves better medical outcomes than its American counterpart. It does so by banning insurance company profits, limiting doctor fees, and accepting shortcomings in care that many well-insured Americans would find intolerable."[6]

Universal and mandatory health care costs the nation 9.6% (2011) of its GDP (slightly over half of what the U.S. spends). It is also less than France or Germany spends on health care, and yet no one can be denied coverage because of pre-existing conditions, or if one becomes bankrupt and unable to pay medical bills. Virtually all aspects of health care are covered (including psychiatric care), although insurance does not pay for some orthodontic work, cosmetic surgeries, and abortions. Strange as it may seem, one has to pay for vaccination. The injuries resulting from drunk accidents are not covered either[7].

The Japanese health care system consists of three major components: Employee's Health Insurance (EHI), National Health Insurance (NHI), and the Citizens Health Insurance Program (CHI).

All companies with 700 or more employees are required to provide their workers with health insurance (EHI). There are 1,800 so–called "society-managed" plans. Quite often a plan covers just one company. People working in small businesses are covered through government run NHI plan. As for the self–employed and retirees, they enroll in municipality run CHI plans.[8]

Enrollment in one of the plans is mandatory and enrollees may not choose a "society-managed" insurance plan that would cover their health expenses: the assignment depends on the employer. The first two insurance programs are financed through payroll deductions. EHI (large companies) deduct 6 to 9.5% of monthly income, of which the employers pay not less than 50% (major corporations may cover as much as 95% of the insurance cost). NHI (small businesses) split the premium: 14% is subsidized by the government; the 86%

balance is deducted from payroll (8.6% of wages), of which employers pay 50%. CHI (the municipal plan) charges the enrollees (depending on income, family size and assets) 0-50% of insurance premiums; the rest is paid by the government. Because the elderly population to be covered by CHI grows disproportionally, all funds contribute to the elderly care.

On average, insurance covers 70% of medical bills. Most Japanese (except for the elderly, the children and those with some chronic disease) have a 30% co-payments. Co-payment of the elderly over the age of 75 and over is 10%; that of children of 3 and younger is 20%. To prevent excessive costs, the government caps co-payments based on patients' income and age. For an average family the cap is about $700 per month; after that they pay just 1%.[6]

In spite of 30% co-payments, only 1% of Japanese purchase supplemental insurance. Annually, a Japanese family spends about $2,500, apart from payroll taxes. Most Japanese are satisfied with their health care system and believe that it is inexpensive.

Like France and Germany, the government imposes a universal fee schedule, which is compulsory for all medical services, including drugs. The reimbursement level of some 3,000 services is set and approved by a 20-member council consisting of representatives of insurance plans, doctors, and medical scientists. Drug prices are also set, and reflect the average market price; preference is given to innovative and more efficient drugs.

Japan has 2.2 practicing physicians per 1,000 population (as of 2011; see the table, in Conclusion). One-third of them work in privately owned clinics, whereas two-thirds are employees of hospitals. Eighty percent of hospitals are private; the most prestigious hospitals are operated by universities. Doctors employed by hospitals have fixed salaries.

In comparison with the U.S., the salaries of hospital doctors are low: on average about $150,000. Doctors are "overworked, overstressed and underpaid."

> Hospital-hired doctors work especially hard. One survey found that 30 percent of them had worked for a month straight without taking any days off . . . Many see dozens of patients a day and are so squeezed for time they do perfunctory examination and don't provide explanations. It is not uncommon for them to take a tip of $1,000 to $2,500 for delivering a baby.[9]

On top of the high patient load they are overwhelmed with paperwork. The most experienced and talented doctors leave hospitals for private (and often quite lucrative) practices: then they earn at least $250,000.

Private clinics often consist of just one doctor without a receptionist or a nurse. Family doctors virtually do not exist in Japan. If there is a medical necessity, people go to any clinic on a first-come first served basis. They may spend 60-75 minutes in a reception room, and just a few minutes with the doctor: "Two-thirds of patients spend less than 10 minutes with their doctor; 18 percent spend less than 3 minutes."[7] It's like an assembly line! Such short visits may be justified because Japanese immediately go to doctors with only a slight suspicion of a problem. The co-payment is insignificant, even though the insurance does not cover the total cost of a doctor visit (and it is typically less than $30, including drugs).[4] On average, a Japanese visits a doctor 13.1 times a year (vs. 4.1 times in the U.S.). Because doctors' fees are fixed, a patient "assembly line" is the only way of making money.[*] I found the claim that "Japanese doctors have more Rolls-Royces than any other profession."[7]

Forty-nine percent of doctors are in primary care: internists, pediatricians, and gynecologists. The rest are specialists, many of them in solo practice. When the problem is serious, the Japanese go to hospitals.

Japan has four times as many hospital beds as the U.S., and a stay is three times longer. Quoting Naohiro Yashiro, a professor and health-care expert at International Christian University in Tokyo:

> Japanese hospitals experience a 'crowding out' effect, with space for emergency care and serious medical conditions sometimes overwhelmed by a flood of patients seeking routine treatment. Patients are treated too equally. Beds are occupied by less urgent cases, and there are no penalties for those who over-use the system."[†4]

Partly as a result of that, even though the Japanese have a lower incidence of heart attacks than Americans, their chances of dying are two times higher.

There is no "gate-keeping" in Japan: no referral to a specialist or a hospital is required. Whereas France and Germany are attempting to implement gate-keeping, Japanese policy-makers are against it. Japan is probably unique: its system is the triumph of moral hazard!

Japanese hospitals experience a deficiency of physicians, especially specialists such as obstetricians, anesthesiologists, and emergency room doctors.

---

[*] Japanese doctors like to prescribe many drugs, partly because their salaries depend on it. It is not uncommon for a single prescription to contain 10 or more drugs. Until recently vitamins were also reimbursable prescription drugs

[†] "Many hospitals have been known to accept 'under the table' payment to see patients quicker. Thus, the market may be working, whether or not policy makers want it to do so." (Ref.[6]).

Hospitals are losing doctors to private practice. Even without moral hazard, the crowding would be quite natural as the number of practicing doctors in Japan (2.2 per 1,000) is significantly lower than in France or Germany (respectively 3.3 and 3.6), where there is no crowding. We in the U.S. also have our own crowding (with 2.5 physicians /1,000): sometimes one has to wait for a specialty doctor appointment for a few weeks). One of the reasons for the scarcity of doctors both in Japan and in the U.S. is the high cost of medical education.

Unlike France and Germany, medical school in Japan is not free. As of 2011, Japan had 80 medical schools (50 national and 30 private).[*] [10] In the least expensive (national) schools in 2006 the annual tuition fee was about $7,000; in a private medical school the average fee was $60,500 and the highest fee was as much as $108,000.[11] Obviously, only affluent families can send their children to private medical schools. Because solo practice is a lucrative business, it is only natural that doctors' children are sent to medical schools, thus creating doctors' "dynasties."

Like in France and Germany, a high school diploma is sufficient to be admitted to a medical school (only 10% of admitted students are college graduates). Undergraduate medical education lasts 6 years: two years of pre-clinical and four years of clinical education. The students pass two national exams after the second and after the sixth year. Postgraduate training takes two years of general residency,[†] and another three or more years of specialty training.[8]

The medical education in Japan lasts 12 years. An 18-year-old high school graduate who enters medical school in Japan doesn't become a full-fledged MD until the age of 30.

Because medical schools in Japan are not free, a Japanese doctor may begin his/her professional life with a significant debt (as in the U.S.). Jichi Medical University has a program that waives the tuition fee if the doctor takes on the obligation to work for 9 years in rural areas. On the other hand, malpractice suits are not as frequent as in the U.S.: less than 1% of physicians are sued, and malpractice insurance is not as expensive as in the U.S. A medical doctor may pay just $500 –$1,000 a year.[‡] The Japanese Medical association covers 45% of doctors, and hospitals carry their doctors' group insurance.[12] The Japanese

---

[*] "Recently [2011], the Japan Medical Association protested the government's desire to increase the number of medical schools as a means of solving the doctor shortage." (*Medical Schools,* 2011. http://blog.japantimes.co.jp/yen-for-living/tag/medical-schools/).

[†] Residents have a reasonable pay, and their work hours are restricted to 40hrs/week (Ref. [9]).

[‡] "Possibly because Japan does not have as many lawyers as the U.S." [sic!]

government suggested creating a program that would automatically pay the patients involved in doctors' errors irrespective of malpractice insurance.[13]

Emergency medical services in Japan[14] are different from those in France and Germany where doctors go to a patient rather than the other way around. The Japanese system is more like the American one, although some elements of the French system are currently being introduced.

Ambulance service is based on fire station paramedics and is the responsibility of local governments. Depending on the seriousness of the case (and some 40% of emergency calls are just another manifestation of moral hazard), paramedics either take the necessary measures to solve the problem or transport the patient to an emergency medical facility.

The average time for ambulance arrival is six minutes, but the transport time may be close to an hour before they find a hospital or a clinic that will accept a patient.[*]

Emergency medical services are provided by emergency hospitals. In various locations, hospitals take turns functioning as "emergency hospitals." They are a part of the "emergency notification system." Sometimes this role is played by "emergency medical care centers" located in regional centers. There also exist the so-called mini-ERs associated with local medical centers or clinics.

In the last ten years, "doctor cars" became a part of the emergency system. After receiving a call requiring a doctor's expertise on site, the doctor leaves the hospital simultaneously with the paramedics and they meet at the patient's location. Because in some (especially rural) areas prompt ambulance service is impossible, a helicopter service is used.

While searching for information on emergency services, I run into sites advertising private emergency services (today in Japan there are 700 private ambulance companies). It is extremely expensive but rather popular, especially among the affluent.

Japan is the fastest aging country in the world, with a low birth rate. Because of the pending deficiency of young working people, in 2003 Japan passed Maternity Leave laws. They are not as liberal as those in France but much more

---

[*] "More than 14,000 emergency patients were rejected at least three times by Japanese hospitals before getting treatment in 2007."
(http://en.wikipedia.org/wiki/Health_care_system_in_Japan). In 2013 "A 75-year-old Japanese man died after 25 hospitals refused to admit him to their emergency rooms 36 times over two hours, citing lack of beds or doctors to treat him."
(http://www.huffingtonpost.com/2013/03/05/japanese-man-dies-after-hospitals-refuse-him_n_2809432.html).

generous than in the U.S.

According to the laws,[15] maternity leave is 14 weeks, usually divided into 6 weeks before and 8 weeks after birth. During the leave the working women typically receive around 40% of their pay (depending on the company). A woman carrying twins is entitled to an additional 8-week leave before giving birth. During the baby's first year, the working mother can take two 30-minute breaks a day to care for her baby. With one month's notice, she can also take a temporary leave. Up to age six the costs of treating children are fully covered.

Compensation for child-care leaves varies from company to company. Large companies are especially generous. In some cases fathers are also eligible for child-care leave. Maternity leave may be extended (for either parent) for one more year. Some companies offer a two- or three-year leave. However, employers do not have to pay the corresponding salaries.

Information about kindergartens in Japan is controversial. There are claims that it is not easy to find good kindergartens and they are expensive. The public day care system is run by municipal governments and the quality of care varies. As I learned from a mother's diary,[16] the children attend kindergarten from around 9 AM till 6 PM; extended stay (till 9:30 PM) is possible with a 10% increased fee. The fee is assigned according to the parents' income. The children have a meal at 11:30 AM, and then a snack after a nap. Children (from toddlers to 5 years old) are divided into small groups (up to 10 children). According to the mother, the care in that nursery is excellent. An interesting detail: diapers are changed every hour, even if they are clean!

Preventive care is a serious business in Japan. Virtually everyone, including foreigners, may have a free health check annually. Companies provide "physicals" to their employees; the self-employed have free or subsidized checks provided by local municipalities. Schoolchildren's examinations are paid for by their schools. Preschoolers and the elderly are under the care of municipalities.[5]

Special attention is paid to women's health. Typically, a woman is informed of her pending mandatory check-up appointment by a local ward government. Her eyes and teeth will be checked, and she will have tests for colon, stomach, and cervical cancer. She will also have a free gynecological examination.[4] According to the Japanese Labor Standards Law, during menstrual period, women are entitled to one day off a month.[*][17] In 2007 the giant company Nike included Menstrual Leave in their Code of Conduct, enforced around the world wherever they operate.

---

[*]Menstrual leave laws exist also in the Philippines, Indonesia and Korea.

Long-term health care (LTC) is an especially important issue in Japan. As I mentioned, Japan has the highest growth of elderly people who may need special medical care. In 2013 the ratio of people over 65 was 24% and is expected to reach 40% by 2060.[18]* Among the elderly, in 2013, 4.62 million had dementia or needed support in fulfilling daily life functions.[19] That number may reach 7.7 million by 2060 – just following the aging of population.

It has been a long–standing tradition in Japan, that family members, especially women, should take care for their parents and parents–in–laws. People still believe that it is a shame on a family to place elderly to nursing homes or use external services for help; "it is akin to abandoning their responsibility as children."[20]

Apart from the moral factor, there are at least three reasons why long-term-care by family members is difficult if not impossible: A family caregiver for an 80+ patient can herself be over 60 years old; an increasingly lesser number of "children" live with the elderly needing LTC (in Tokyo it dropped below 50%); an increasingly larger number of women work for a living and are unable to help.

To meet this problem, the Public Long-Term Care Insurance Law was implemented in 2000.[†18] Its main objective has been to shift the burden of caring for the elderly from the family to qualified medical personnel either at home or in special institutions. This law encourages expanding LTC from the public to the private sector.

The public LTC program is funded through taxes, and an individual's fee (0-100%) depends on many factors. Among them are the income of the patient and his/her family members and the number of relations who are able to contribute to LTC. A co-payment is also necessary: one has to pay up to 10% of the insurance cost (in a nursing facility a meal co-pay also applies). For people below the poverty line health care is free.

Hospitals in Japan are readily accessible. Therefore many elderly people chose admission to a hospital rather than welfare system with complex check of incomes and family situation. This is a so-called "social hospitalization," which uses as many as 15% of hospital beds.[21] And this is in spite of the fact that staying in a hospital is 1.8 times more expensive than staying in a nursing

---

* The U.S. will achieve that rate only in some 125 years! By 2050, 20% of our population will be older than 65. (http://www.census.gov/population/www/pop-profile/elderpop.html).
† This is the fifth social insurance program in Japan after medical care insurance, pension insurance, unemployment and occupational accident compensation insurance.

home. Simply because of nursing home's severe shortage.

Welfare services: both at home and in special facilities (such as nursing homes) are provided and regulated by municipalities. After taking into account family's income and general condition, they decide which services should be provided, and to what extend. Low-income people have a higher priority, comparing with middle income ones.

Here are the total LTC insurance benefits:[18]
Home Care Services:
• Nurse visit and home care aid (24 hours including at night in case of need)
• Rehabilitation service at home and day-care center
• Medical management
• Respite care services
• Day care center services
• Group home service for seniors with dementia
• Home visiting bathing service (mobile bathtub)
• Home care devices (wheelchair, special beds, etc.)
• Minor home remodeling (eliminating steps, installing handrails, etc.)
Institutional Services:
• Special nursing homes for the elderly
• Health service facilities for the elderly
• Geriatric care hospitals (long-term care ward)

In 2005 the total cost of LTC insurance was over $70 million and the individual monthly premium was $35. In 2010 the total cost exceeded $85 million, and the individual payment was $45/month.[18]

Japan is an Eastern country with deeply implanted ancient traditions. Especially strong is the influence of ancient Chinese philosophy based on Confucian ideas.[*] As a natural consequence, alternative medicine based on Chinese traditions is very popular and its popularity is increasing tremendously.

The sale of herbal and Chinese medications in 2008 exceeded $200 million. Especially popular are herbal medications that claim to burn fat. One hundred

---

[*] "Confucian ethics give Japanese family relations a special flavor. Indeed . . . owing to traditional Confucian ideas, family-based support receives special emphasis in the social welfare programs of Japan and East Asian countries. Thanks to such indigenous factors, Japanese family policies may appear as distinct from those in European countries, irrespective of economic and demographic convergence."(http://www.ipss.go.jp/webj-ad/WebJournal.files/population/2003_6/2.Fukuda.pdf).

forty six herbal drugs are covered by public insurance. Among the traditional Japanese medicines are *gennoshoko* (Japanese geranium), an effective treatment for diarrhea and digestive infections; *dokudami*, a low creeping plant with white flowers and a nasty smell used to treat heart problems and counteract poisons; *ukon* (turmeric), which helps the liver and fights bacteria; and feverfew (bachelor's button, or *natsushirogiku*), a popular relief for migraine headaches. Some questionable medicines include *sumi*, snakes roasted on a stick until black, which are added to food as a general tonic.

(Those interested, I direct to a University of Maryland website on Japanese herbal medicine[22])

Massage, acupuncture, and Shiatsu are very popular in Japan.[*] Children are taught to give neck and shoulder massage to their fathers after a difficult day at work.

Japan has one of the most powerful economies in the world. No wonder that technologically, Japan's health care system is well ahead of other developed countries. Over 70% of Japanese hospitals have whole-body CT-scanners and 30% of hospitals have MRI machines. According to OECD data (see the table in Conclusion), the number of MRI/CT units per million population is the world highest: 43.1/97.3 compared to 31.6/40.0 in the U.S. In comparison with Canada, France, and Germany, Japanese health care has some unique features. No wonder! Japan is a unique country with strong traditions and the highest life expectancy in the world: 85.9 years for women and 79.4 for men, and one of the lowest child mortality rates: 2.3 deaths/1,000 births (see the table in Conclusion).

Over 80% of Japanese people are satisfied with their health care system. However, the main reason for its low cost is that doctors, nurses and other medical personnel working for hospitals are severely underpaid, whereas the solo clinic specialists are Rolls-Royce rich due to "assembly lines," in which patients participate for an insignificant fee and co-pay. The Japanese smoke a lot: in Japan there are 500,000 cigarette vending machines, in spite of the fact that smoking is among the main causes of death. And yet, the anti-smoking propaganda and anti-smoking laws are weak.

The Japanese are less obese than Americans. And yet for 70 percent of population there is a compulsory obesity screening. In case one is found to be fat around the waist, he/she is required to attend counseling and begin an exercise program and diet.[4] If anybody would dare to implement such a measure in the U.S, libertarians would issue a call to arms to defend the freedom to be fat.

---

[*] Professional massagers and acupuncturists are traditionally blind people.

As I mentioned, Japan provides a free annual check-up to almost all its citizens and even to foreigners. Such preventive measures don't seem all that necessary because people have a healthy lifestyle, and do not get sick often; there is less crime and fewer car accidents. In spite of liking to stay in hospitals, people in general oppose invasive procedures. The nation's intrinsic good health is one of the factors that makes Japanese health care less expensive than it is in France (9.6% of GDP vs. 11.6%), while Israel spends on health care even less –7.7% GDP.

However, the Japanese economy is in a deep crisis and has been for a long time. The population is rapidly aging: 40% will be 65 and older in 2055. Diseases that are more costly to treat (among them cancer, stroke and Alzheimer's) are becoming more frequent. Within the next 25 years the demand (and the cost) for medical care will increase threefold.

Fortunately, the Japanese health care system is in a state of permanent reform, attempting to cut costs with minimal decrease in quality. One may hope that its positive features and advantages will not be sacrificed.

United Kingdom

The United Kingdom (the U.K.), or Britain, or England, is short for the official name: The United Kingdom of Great Britain and Northern Ireland. Administratively, the U.K. is divided into four regions: England, Northern Ireland, Scotland, and Wales. Each of them has its own government. The U.K. is a constitutional monarchy. Its parliament consists of the House of Lords and the House of Commons. Queen Elizabeth II is the nominal head of state. She appoints the Prime Minister (head of the party that has the largest number of seats in the House of Commons) and approves candidates for government posts. Great Britain has not accepted the EURO as its monetary system, and still uses the Pound Sterling (£). As of May 2014, £1=$1.68.

The "Great Britain" in the country's official name is the name of the island. Obviously, this name is nostalgic. In the nineteenth and the beginning of the twentieth century Britain was *Great*: the British Empire was the largest empire that world history knew. In 1922, after the end of World War I and the destruction of the Ottoman Empire, Great Britain ruled over one fifth of the earth's land surface and a quarter of its population. It was said that the sun never sets on the British Empire!

What is left of the Empire is the *British Commonwealth* – an organization of 54 independent states, 52 of which had been part of the British Empire (the largest are Canada, Australia and India). The ceremonial head of the Commonwealth is Queen Elizabeth; she is also the monarch of 16 Commonwealth states (Canada, Australia and New Zealand are among them).

Today Britain occupies the island of Great Britain, a part of Northern Ireland, which Britain shares with the Republic of Ireland, and a number of small islands. Associated with the U.K. are also three crown dependencies and fourteen overseas territories.

In spite of the loss of a quarter of the world, England is still a great nation culturally, scientifically, politically, economically, and militarily. She is also a member of the "nuclear club." Her GDP is the sixth largest in the world.

The English National Health System (NHS) was born on July 5, 1948. It was based on three principles: [1]

-It meets the needs of everyone
-Its delivery is free
-It is based on clinical need and not the ability to pay.

As I mentioned in the introduction to this chapter, the NHS is known as the Beveridge system. The First Baron William Beveridge was an active proponent of public health care. When the New World emerged from the destruction of World War II, he saw such a system as crucial for slaying the five giants: "want, disease, squalor, ignorance, and idleness."[2] It seems that over 60 years later those giants have only gained more power and are now threatening our civilization.

The NHS is the largest public health system in the world and the largest single-payer system.[2] It employs more than 1.5 million people. "Only Wal-Mart, the Indian Railways, and the Chinese People's Liberation Army directly employ more people than the NHS."[1]

Functionally, the NHS is subdivided into two sectors: Primary and Secondary care. Primary care (PC) is the frontline of the NHS: it is the first point of contact of a patient with the system. PC is delivered by general practitioners, optometrists, dentists, and pharmacists who may be independent contractors. Secondary Care (SC), sometimes called "Acute Health care," is the second line of defense: specialists, hospitals, and emergency care. The NHS literally delivers health care for all.[3]

Anyone who is legitimately registered with the system (i.e., has an NHS number), both UK citizens and also legal immigrants, has access to the full scope of medical care without any out-of-pocket payment of any kind. In this respect the NHS is, probably, unique.

Tourists, temporary workers, and illegal immigrants are not eligible for all medical services. However, emergency care is provided free of charge to everyone, regardless of legal status or citizenship. Actually, it is like a world service: "anyone on the planet can theoretically take advantage, provided they are able to physically enter the country first[*]"

Although England spends only 9.4% of its GDP on health care (compared with the U.S.'s 17.6%), the NHS costs the government 15.6% of its budget.

The NHS is financed mostly by general taxation (about 90%). However, in England, Wales, Scotland, and Northern Ireland the NHS is administered separately. Each of the four provinces has its own tax income and budget. The money is transferred to trusts. The Primary Care Trust consumes 80% of the NHS's budget.

England's tax system is relatively simple (compared, say, with that of France or Germany). Everyone has a Personal Allowance (in the U.S. we call it standard deduction). In 2012-2013 this allowance for people under 65 and income below $180,000, was $13,600 (in 2011-2012 it was $ 13,000); married couples, the elderly, the blind and some other categories of citizens have an increased PA. Those who earn less than PA do not pay taxes. Income above the PA is taxed at 20% up to $52,300; at 40% over this amount up to $240,000; and at 45% on income over $240,000.[4]

Another source of the government's budget is the National Insurance Contribution that is paid by all employed and the self-employed, and which covers state pensions, unemployment benefits, and some other allowances. Based on weekly earnings, the NIC is withheld from the regular income of employees and the self-employed, with the employers' contribution of 12.8%. On average, the NIC amounts to an additional 20% of a middle bracket gross income (and brings the marginal tax bracket to 58%).[5] Like everywhere in Europe, the English also pay the VAT (Value Added Tax) of 20% on virtually any purchase. It is actually a consumption tax, which discourages purchasing anything that is not truly necessary. Such a tax in the U.S. would bring about a recession.

As I mentioned, primary care is the core of NHS, and its foundation is the army of thirty-five thousand general practitioners (GPs) comprising 30 percent of all physicians (see the Table in the concluding chapter). GPs play an important role in any health care system. Upon careful examination of a patient and after

---

[*] Anonymous blogger.

compiling a detailed anamnesis, an experienced GP can correctly diagnose about 85% of health problems. The remaining 15% may need a consultation with a specialist. In England the GP is the gate-keeper to the acute care realm: specialists, hospital consultations and procedures. One cannot enter that gate without a GP's referral. However, one does not need a referral to see dentists, pharmacists, and optometrists.

GPs (and other primary care doctors) are independent contractors. The government (Primary Care Trust) gives GPs a definite basic sum of money depending on the number of patients they see (their numbers are known because everybody covered by the NHS has his/her GP). What is important: a GP's budget depends on the number of registered patients, no matter whether they attend his/her office that year or not. This is a power stimulus for doctors to keep their patients healthy, so that they attend his office as infrequently as possible!

Doctors earn additional bonuses depending on experience and the quality of care they provide. Every GP has to accumulate a certain number of quality points that are crucial in establishing the next year's budget. Dr. Nigel Hawkes, MD, a health editor for *The Times of London* said in an interview:

> The quality points are things like making sure you've tracked down everybody in your practice who's got diabetes or heart disease, and you've treated them appropriately, and you've kept in touch with them, and you've called them every six months, those kind of things.[6]

Quality bonuses can reach a third of the GP's budget. It is not clear how the number of quality points the GP earns, based on his/her judgment, can be controlled. At least this is a kind of "market" mechanism of improving the quality of health care. And the government continuously reformulates quality points making it more difficult to acquire the maximum possible number.

From the budget that the GP receives, he/she pays for the set-up of the practice (typically shared by a few doctors and other medical and clerical personnel) and all expenses; what is left is his/her annual income.

A patient may choose a GP he/she likes, and can switch to a different doctor without restrictions if, of course, a GP who accepts new patients is available locally. All such changes have to be registered with the local authorities.

Whereas GPs are free-lance contractors (although paid by government), most specialty doctors work for hospitals. The Hospital Trust defines budgets for all non-private hospitals. The hospitals' budgets (apart from the salaries of their employees) are based on government "tariffs," (e.g., delivering a baby costs $1,500; an amputation – $10,500; hip replacement – $11,500). However, in no way do these tariffs affect surgeons' or other medical personnel's salaries. They are set by categories, depending on the experience of the doctor/nurse. Strange as it may seem, a specialist's salary in a hospital is not much larger than a GP's income. Like GPs, specialists can also earn quality points, called "Clinician Excellence Points," which affect doctors' promotions to higher pay categories.

GPs are easily accessible within 1 to 3 days. To see a specialist ("consultant") is a different story. The GP issues a referral to a particular specialist. The patient may request a referral to a different specialist if there are convincing reasons for this request. Upon booking the appointment, the patient is placed in a queue. It is not on last-come-last-served basis; the queue depends on the urgency of appointment. For a non-urgent specialist appointment or surgery the median wait time is 6 weeks. The maximum wait time is 18 weeks.[7]

England is also infamous for long wait times for diagnostic services. The wait time for MRI, CT scan, ultrasound examination, colonoscopy, and other diagnostic procedures may be as long as six weeks. Especially dangerous is the long wait time for diagnosing cancer.

The government "Operational Standards for the Cancer Waiting Times Commitments"[8] issued in 2005–2009 and still working today "standardized" the maximal wait time for cancer treatment:

> Two Week Wait Standard - In addition to all patients with suspected cancer, all patients referred with any breast symptoms should have their first hospital appointment with 14 days (two weeks) of the referral being received at the hospital even if cancer is not suspected.

> 31 Day Standard- The 31 Day Standard now applies to all cancers, irrespective of whether they are new or recurrent, relapsed or metastatic. In addition all surgical and drug therapy treatments (not just first treatment) will be subject to a 31 Day Standard, e.g. a patient receiving surgery post radiotherapy must receive their surgery within 31 days of the decision to treat surgically being made.

> 31 Day Standard- All subsequent treatments (not just surgery and drug therapy) will be subject to the 31 Day Standard, so every new and subsequent treatment will need to be delivered within one month (31 days) of a decision to treat date or an 'earliest clinically appropriate date'

> 62 Day Standard- The 62 Day Standard now applies to referrals from National Screening Services (Bowel, Cervical and Breast screening). So patients diagnosed with a cancer that has been detected via the screening program will need to start their treatment within 62 days of the screening referral.

One can see that a month can pass between a diagnosis and the beginning of treatment. I could not find any explanations for this. The long queues most probably are primarily the result of the shortage of doctors and sophisticated equipment. England has a total of 2.8 physicians per 1000 population (against 3.8 in Germany, and 3.3 in France and Israel). The main shortage of doctors is among specialists and young ("junior;" see below) doctors, although the number of specialists is twice that of GPs. The U.S. has 2.5 doctors per 1000 population, but such wait times are unheard of here, especially for cancer treatment.

The shortage of equipment (MRI machines, CT scans, etc.) has probably the same origin as in Canada: the government does not have enough funds to purchase such equipment. The U.K. has 5.9 MRI machines and 8.2 CT scanners per million population, whereas in the U.S. it is 31.6 and 40. (See the table in Conclusion.)

In order to avoid long wait times and be assured of better service quality, 11.5% of Britons purchase private health insurance, which supplements the NHS.

It is not easy to estimate how much a GP makes. As a freelance doctor, the GP's income often depends on his/her entrepreneurial talent. According to the official data,[9] in 2011-2012 an average gross earning of a GP working for Primary Medical Services was $504,000. This is the government's salary that probably includes both basic pay and bonuses. Subtracting expenses ($321,000), the net income comes to $183,000. However, a GP can earn much more if he/she finds time for private practice.

Specialists (in England named "consultants") are mostly employees of hospitals and earn according to hospitals' pay scales. Both the base salaries and quality bonuses depend on the doctor's experience. The basic pay for 0 to 18 years of experience is $111,700 to $150,000. If we add bonuses ($4,500 to $100,000), we arrive at the fork $116,000 to $250,000. Again, a consultant can earn more through private practice. As one can see, on average, a GP makes more money than a young, inexperienced specialist.

Medical education in England is four years shorter than in the U.S. Like in France, Germany and Japan, to be admitted to a medical school one does not need a bachelor's degree. A high-school diploma is sufficient.

However, an applicant has to have virtually all As on graduation exams. Those who intend to go to university have to pass extremely difficult A-Level exams.[*]

England has 32 medical schools. The competition to be accepted to a school is fierce. Some medical schools require passing special entrance exams. Undergraduate medical education takes five years and awards the degrees of Bachelor of Medicine and Bachelor of Surgery (BMBS). Although these are two separate degrees, they are awarded simultaneously. This undergraduate education gives both basic medical knowledge and teaches some clinical and diagnostic skills. However, the basic medical education also requires two years of so-called foundation training (what we in the U.S. call residency) in hospitals: F1 and F2:

The F1 includes three months of general surgery and three months of general medicine, with the other six months made up of work in other areas of specialist interest.

The F2 consists of three four-month placements and includes opportunities to work in primary care as well as developing core skills in time management, IT and team working.

Until one is licensed in a definite specialty, one is called a *junior doctor*. F1 and F2 trainings are the beginning of a doctor's career. To become a GP, one has to work under supervision for another three years (total time in training is five years). To become a specialist the total training time is a minimum of 8 years.[10] A junior doctor's salary varies from approximately $50,000 a year (F1 and F2) to $75,000 after five years of specialist training.

In 2010 England had to accept the European Union's regulation that a medical resident did not have to work more than 48 hours a week. This decision was controversial: residents were displeased because their salaries dropped almost 40% (working over 48 hours a week means well-paid overtime); hospital administrators were displeased because they now needed more doctors, even though medical mistakes decreased because the load on overworked residents diminished.

Medical school undergraduate education (five years) is not free: typically it costs about $5,000 a year (plus living expenses). Thus, upon graduation, a junior doctor has a debt of $40,000 – $100,000[11] (lodging and food are quite expensive in England), which is significantly less than the debt a young U.S.

---

[*] The late Dr. John Silber, a noted educator and former president of Boston University, wrote in his 1989 book *Straight Shooting: What Is Wrong With America And How To Fix It*: "At the present moment, I believe very few [American] college graduates could pass the A-Level examinations required in England of students who wish merely to enter the university."

doctor faces.

As I mentioned, every person on English soil is eligible for free emergency services. When one calls the emergency number (999), the wait time for an ambulance depends on the type of emergency. For Category A (life-threatening) emergencies the official target is 19 minutes. For Category B: non-life-threatening (though serious) emergencies, the wait time may be much longer. In 2011 the 19-minute target was replaced by a range of indicators including "time to treatment"[12] (they won't be rushing to get there in 19 minutes for a nosebleed).

When the patient is brought to an ER (in Britain they are called A&E: Accident and Emergency room), one has to be prepared for long wait. The target of a doctor's response to Category A patients is 8 minutes. Until 2011, the maximum waiting time was set by the government at four hours. Now this target remains the same for accidents and emergencies but in other situations, as Andrew Lansley, the former Health Secretary, said, "The new measures will focus on quality of care and what matters most to patients - giving a better indication of patient care than the previous process-led targets ever could,"[12] which means that some other quality measures in an emergency situation may be more important than the doctor's immediate response. (Americans are used to "innovations" like that, the only true meaning of which is *expect that things will get worse.**)

In England, approximately 800,000 malpractice events occur each year. However, only 1% of them become the subject of a claim and even those rarely go to court.

English doctors do not practice "defensive medicine" in American sense: conducting tests and procedures even if they are not necessary. Their defense is that every procedure or test appropriate for a given diagnosis is listed in government instructions. It is, actually, like a "check-list." If the doctor has fulfilled all the formalized requirements, he/she virtually cannot be accused of malpractice. A wrong diagnosis, followed by a string of wrong procedures and

---

* The political situation in today's England (2013) is quite strained. David Cameron, the leader of the conservative party has initiated a number of measures directed at cutting government spending, primarily on the NHS. Naturally, the left-wing media is against these measures. As a result, time and again I have come across articles (say, in *The Guardian*) exaggerating the consequences of those measures and even presenting inaccurate figures. I have to check and re-check most of them. As for people who share in blogs their responses to the increasing rationing of their medical services, most of them defend their system while acknowledging that changes are needed.

medication, is a different story.

If a doctor is employed by a hospital, the hospital deals with malpractice claims and pays when necessary. The GPs (as well as other PC physicians: dentists, pharmacists, optometrists and other self-employed professionals) are on their own: they are not covered by the government.

They usually belong to unions or medical defense societies, which render assistance in malpractice situations. As for the insurance premiums, they are quite low: a GP may pay under $1,000 a year, less than one tenth of what an American doctor pays.

Maternity leave.[13] A working woman in England has a 52-week statutory maternity leave: "Ordinary Maternity leave" (first 26 weeks), and "Additional Maternity Leave" (last 26 weeks). The woman does not have to take all 52 weeks, but must take two weeks after baby is born. Thirty-nine weeks of maternity leave are paid: 90% of her regular salary for the first 6 weeks, and $225 weekly for the remaining 33 weeks. Another 13 weeks are unpaid. A pregnant woman may request the beginning of her paid leave 11 weeks before the baby is to be born. During the statutory leave the woman may not be fired, and after it ends she returns to her original position and pay.

The woman's husband or partner (irrespective of sex) is also eligible for a 26-week parental leave, of which two weeks are paid weekly at $225.

The baby's delivery may take place either in a hospital or at home. It is supervised by a midwife, unless a doctor's presence is necessary. Typically, the woman is discharged from hospital within a few hours after delivery. A midwife (either the same who assisted at the delivery or a different one) will visit the baby regularly at home between 10 and 28 days after the baby is born.

Day-to-day care for children's health is provided by a network of Sure Start Children's Centers.[14] In 2013, there were over 3000 such centers in England. The centers are staffed with experienced physicians and nurses who provide treatments for common children's illnesses that do not require hospitalization, such as infections or diarrhea and also periodic health-checks and vaccinations.

Children's free education begins at the age of three.[15] Nursery school attendance at ages three and four is not mandatory. Mandatory education begins at the age of five and ends at 16. In order to be eligible to enter a university, two more years of study (called "sixth form") are required. These are typically completed with Class A examinations.

Like in every developed country in the world, England's population is aging. Today over 10 million people are older than 65; that number will reach 12 million in 2020. Their health care accounts for about 70% of total health-care spending. The elderly often use their GPs disproportionately (50% of appointments), and take up 60% to 70% of hospitals' capacities.

Long-term health care (LTC) in England (it is called "continuing care") has a complicated structure.[16] It is partly supported from public funds (the NHS and local authorities), but the larger percentage is paid by the elderly or their families. Means testing ("the meanest means testing!") places an assets limit, above which public support dwindles. As of 2011 that limit was about $35,000, which includes savings, investments, and may also include the value of the elderly person's home. NHS assistance stops at that limit, although local authorities may partly subsidize LTH care, depending on the patient's assets. Below approximately $19,000 (depending on the province), coverage is complete.

The NHS takes care of LTH care (medical, not social) outside hospitals or nursing homes, such as home care (personal care and care of the house). Additional care may be provided by private helpers (a typical pay to helpers is $15/hour).

There is a variety of assisted living options, of which the NHS covers only the medical part (possibly restricted because of the asset limitation). Additional financial help is provided by local authorities (councils) from their own budgets. There is an asset requirement that in many cases cuts off the subsidies.

Nursing homes (called "care homes") are quite expensive in England. On average, they cost between $50,000 and $75,000/year ($140 to $200/day).* Care homes provide basic personal needs (meals, bathing), as well as nursing care. Although the NHS does not pay for the basic care, it does pay for the services of certified nurses ($165/week).

As one can see, the elderly middle class should think about financing its LTC. The low assets threshold results in fast pauperization of the elderly who eventually have to sell their homes in order to pay LTC expenses and eventually become 100% eligible for government support.† Whereas 11.5% of the English purchase private health insurance supplementing the NHS, only 2% purchase private LTH insurance. There is a kind of denial among the aging English that they *must* contribute to their LTH expenditure: About 40% of British adults believe they should not have to pay for social and nursing care in

---

* For comparison, tuition in Eaton, one of the most prestigious private schools, costs about $45,000/year.
† Does this not remind us of the situation with LTH in the U.S.? In order to pay for a nursing home people exhaust all their savings and eventually become eligible for Medicaid, Like Americans, the English also attempt to hide their assets in order to look poor.

retirement.

In 2013 a government commission, Fairer Care Funding, put forward a proposal that will make it easier for people to pay for LTC.[17] To begin with, a life-time cap on the maximum from pocket spending will be established: about $120,000. Financial support by government will be available for people with assets up to about $195,000 (up from about $40,000 before). People will have to pay nursing home living expenses. Those living in their homes will have to pay living expenses up to about $20,000 a year. Also, a universal deferred payment scheme that will prevent people from selling their homes to cover residential care.

This is quite a radical reform suggestion. If approved by the Parliament, it will become a law from 2016. Close to concluding my story of England's health care, I am ambivalent, as most of my readers will probably be. The English health care system, though it provides everybody with good care, is strongly centralized, and, therefore, bureaucratized.

Thus far I have not mentioned an important arm of the NHS: the National Institute for Health and Care (formerly Clinical) Excellence, or NICE. NICE issues "Clinical Guidelines And Recommendations On The Appropriate Treatment And Care Of People With Specific Diseases And Conditions Within the NHS In England And Wales,"[*][18] which means that its main function is to

decide which treatments doctors may use, and which medicines may be approved for these treatments. Although NICE controls the quality of health care, its main objective is to adjust medical treatment to the available funds, which is actually rationing. Quite a few drugs have become unavailable because of their high price.[1] Under scrutiny is also the rationing of spending on the final stage of people's lives. NICE estimated that the ceiling of spending in the last 6 months of life was $50,000 ("but exceptions are made").[2] What both the "ceiling" and the "exceptions" mean are not clear...Do the English like their health care system? Some do and some don't. I saw, on blogs, statements like: "I pay 1/3 of my income to health care, and don't have to bother," and "Why don't we, the Brits, go to the streets and protest this behemoth of inefficient health care of ours?" Of course, decades of being a welfare state strongly instilled a dependency mentality in people's psyches. I do not think this is a lesson American health care reformers should learn.

---

[*] An earlier version of the President Obama's PPACA reform required creation of the *Federal Coordinating Council for Comparative Effectiveness Research*, which, according to some interpretations, would have more–or–less the same functions: it would encourage bureaucratic interference with physicians' decision-making. It was removed from the most recent Bill.

Being an optimist, I am sure that the English system will gradually change into a more flexible, less welfarish one. After conservatives have come to power, some changes are already noticeable. My worry is, however, that England, like most European countries, may not have much time for any changes before succumbing to Muslimezation.

Israel

Israel (*Medinat Israel* in Hebrew) is the only state in the world created "from scratch." It came into being in 1948 by virtue of the United Nations decision. Israel is a democratic nation – a tiny piece of land surrounded by hostile, totalitarian Arab states. Out of the total population of 8,132,000 (January, 2014), 6,102,000 (75.2%) are Jewish, the balance are the Arabs, 1,682,000 (20.6%), the Druze, 130,000 (1.6%), and other minorities.[3]

Israel has a complex political system, at the top of which is a Prime Minister – the head of the party having the largest representation in the Knesset, the unicameral Parliament consisting of 120 members. The formal head of State,

the President, plays only a symbolic role. Israel has the Basic Law – a substitute for a Constitution.[*]

The currency of Israel is the New Israeli Shekel (NIS). As of May 2014, NIS1.

---

[*] One of the reasons for the absence of Constitution is that Israel has a high percentage (about 25%) of Orthodox religious Jews (8%-ultra-orthodox, and 17% – "modern orthodox" or religious Zionists) who play a significant role in political life; 55% are "traditionalists," who adhere to some religious commandments, and 20% are secular (http://www.jcpa.org/dje/articles2/relinisr-consensus.htm). In Israel there is no separation of religion and state. As a result of "ideological diversity" (and too often intransigence – and not only between the religious and the secular) there is no consensus of the nation's "status." Is it a "democratic republic" or a realization of G-d's Promise to gather the Jews into the Holy Land? On top of that, since her establishment, Israel has not have stable and internationallyacknowledged borders. All this poses serious obstacles to devising formal judicial statements regarding the nature of the State, based on general consensus with religious parties. To say nothing of the fact that there are ultra-orthodox anti-Zionist groups; among them *Neturei Karta* whose members refuse to recognize the existence and authority of the State of Israel, which must not have been created before coming of the Ha Mashiach (Messia).

Who Cares about Health Care?

= $0.29.

Today Israel has a highly developed high-tech–dominated economy. Within a decade Israel may become a high-tech superpower.

In his 2009 Cairo speech, President Obama said that "the aspiration for a Jewish homeland is rooted in a tragic history," implying that Israel is the place where Jews who survived the Holocaust (the murder of 6 million Jews by the Nazis) eventually found their home, hinting at the similarity between the Jews as "refugees" and the Arab refugees. Although this book is not the place for arguing the legitimacy of Israel (which is now being questioned throughout the world), I want to mention the lamentation in Psalm 137:5:

"If I forget thee oh Jerusalem, let my right arm wither . . ."

which was written by a Jewish poet some 2,500 years ago in Babylonian exile. Return to Zion and Jerusalem had always been the powerful dream of a hundred generations of Jews. Whenever Israelis mention leaving or returning to Israel, they use the word Eretz–the *Land*.

For my readers who are unfamiliar with the *true* history of Israel (as opposed to numerous myths created in the recent 60+ years), I recommend informative sources.[4] Just a few facts here, without which it would be impossible to understand the Israeli health-care system.

Jewish immigration to Eretz never ceased during the two millennia. The idea of rebuilding a Jewish home in Palestine, spurred by Zionist movement (born at the end of the 19th century) significantly enhanced immigration. At that time Palestine, a desolate, barren land, was under the rule of the Turkish Ottoman Empire. In World War I Turkey was defeated and Palestine became a mandate territory governed by Great Britain.

In 1917, a century after the Jewish immigration to Eretz Israel became popular among European Jews, Britain approved "in principle", with the Balfour Declaration, the establishment of a "Jewish Homeland" in Palestine. However, in its practical policy, Britain did whatever was possible to prevent the resettlement of Jews in Palestine.

After the defeat of the Nazis when their genocide of Jews became known to the world, the newly born United Nations, under pressure from a majority of member states, voted to partition Palestine into a Jewish state and an Arab state in 1947. After the last British soldier left on May 14, 1948, the State of Israel was officially announced by David Ben Gurion, the Head of the World Zionist Organization (which was an official representative of the Jewish population, "the Yishuv").

On the very next day, the armies of six Arab countries invaded the young

Jewish state. However, the Arab armies were crushed! To some it was a "miracle" (with quotation marks or without)[*]: The cease-fire on Jan. 7, 1949, established new Israeli borders, which included 50% more land than had been contained in the original partition. However, East Jerusalem was lost to the Jews and was returned to Israel only during the Six Day War in 1967.

The first waves of *chalutzim* – the Jewish settlers – were mostly educated people with a socialist ideology. They wanted to work on land and founded communal agricultural settlements, *kibbutzim*. The land was barren; the settlers had to drain swamps, plant woods, and make earth available for agriculture. And this is under permanent threat of Arab's attacks.

established new Israeli borders, which included 50% more land than had been contained in the original partition. However, East Jerusalem was lost to the Jews and was returned to Israel only during the Six Day War in 1967.

---

[*] The history of Israel is a succession of events that look like miracles. The first "miracle" happened decades before the creation of the State of Israel. At the end of the 19th century the Jewish settlers communicated mostly in Yiddish and other dialects from "old countries." Through the enthusiasm and energy of *one* person, Eliezer Ben-Yehuda (who emigrated to Eretz Israel in 1881), Hebrew, which had been used before only as a sacred language in prayers and Judaic studies, became the official language of the nation. The second "miracle" was the creation of the State in 1948. It would not have happened had Stalin decided to veto the UN resolution, and Truman succumbed to the anti-Jewish pressure of his administration. Later, the Soviet Union became Israel's worst enemy, arming and training terrorists. ("The term "Palestinian People" as a descriptive of Arabs in Palestine appeared for the first time in the preamble of the 1964 PLO Charter, drafted in Moscow": http://www.think-israel.org/ brand.russiatheenemy.html). The third "miracle" was the victory of Israel, outnumbered by Arab armies 100:1, in the first war (1948-1949); it appeared to be impossible, but it happened. I would like to mention one more event of a miraculous proportion. It was the immigration to Israel of a million Soviet Jews during two decades: the nineteen-eighties and nineteen-nineties. At that time there was a joke: if an immigrant getting off a plane at Ben-Gurion Airport did not carry a violin or a cello case, then that person was a pianist. However, apart from the enormous cultural infusion that the new immigrants brought to Israel, they brought their scientific and technical knowledge. And they brought their children, who had been refused acceptance to Soviet universities. Israel has been able (albeit with great difficulty) to absorb this army of talent that has changed the face of the nation. Today Israel has the largest number of high-tech and biomedical start-up companies per capita. And I would like to mention one more "miracle": the resurrection of the Jewish *nation* out of a number of culturally and ethnically different pieces, including black Ethiopian Jews, who are now full-fledged Israeli citizens.

Who Cares about Health Care?

The first waves of *chalutzim* – the Jewish settlers – were mostly educated people with a socialist ideology. They wanted to work on land and founded communal agricultural settlements, *kibbutzim*. The land was barren; the settlers had to drain swamps, plant woods, and make earth available for agriculture. And this is under permanent threat of Arab's attacks.

To provide basic health care, and fight diseases such as dysentery, malaria, typhus and trachoma, which were rampant in the 19th century, a few clinics and hospitals were organized, mostly in large cities.

Thus, the foundation of the current health system was laid well before the state was created, both before and during the period of British Mandate (1918-1948). By the time of the establishment of the State of Israel a health care infrastructure was already in place and successfully functioning.

In 1911 the first Jewish insurance company, *Kupat Holim Clalit* ("General Sick Fund"), was organized and later taken over by the Histadrut (the General Federation of Labor, a politically powerful union). Before the creation of the State, three other Sick Funds (SFs): *Kupat Holim Maccabi*, *Kupat Holim Meuhedet* and *Kupat Holim Leumit*, which continue to function today, were also organized. By the end of 1948, only 53% of Israelis carried health insurance, and 80% of those were insured by the Clalit.[5]

Before 1995 the SFs had strong political affiliations and were more than just sick funds: they sponsored youth organizations, sports clubs, and so on. Enrollment in Clalit – the arm of the powerful Histadrut – was mandatory for workers belonging to this union (and virtually everybody belonged). After 1995 political affiliations were prohibited, and the Clalit enrollment today has dropped to only half of the population.

In 1995 the National Health-Care Law was passed by the Knesset; it is now the foundation of Israel's well-functioning high-standard health-care system.

The 2000 WHO ranking put Israel as No. 28 (out of 190 nations), between the United Arab Emirates (No. 27) and Morocco (No. 29). This ranking has been criticized for its politicization. However, in four categories out of five Israel was ranked rather high. As we will see, the accusation of Israeli health care in "inequity" by the WHO rating is unfair. The more objective 2013 Bloomberg ratings that I mentioned in the Introduction to this chapter elevated Israel to No. 4 in system efficiency, and No. 6 in health care quality.

According to the National Health-Care Law, all Israel's permanent residents must have health insurance through one of the four above-mentioned non-profit SFs: Kupat Holim Clalit (the largest), Kupat Holim Maccabi, Kupat Holim Meuhedet, and Kupat Holim Leumit. All SFs are self-ruled. Government regulations are restricted only to formulating and enforcing the rules the SFs operate under and distributing funds. For example, the cost of insurance is the same in all four SFs.

Israelis are free to join any SF and can switch to a different one every six months (only 1% of people actually do). SFs are Health Management Organizations (HMOs): they have their own clinics, preferred hospitals, and preferred physicians. However, private doctors and clinics typically accept payment from SFs.

Upon enrolling in an SF, a patient is assigned a primary care physician (PCP), who is easily accessible, and the visits are free. In order to see a specialist, the patient needs a PCP's referral to a physician affiliated with the SF (or a private doctor), although some specialists such as gynecologists, pediatricians, ophthalmologists, and some others (depending on the SF) do not require referrals. Upon visiting a specialist one has a co-pay of about $6.50 once in a quarter.

SFs compete with each other. This is called "regulated competition." People are attracted to a definite SF or decide to stay away from another SF based on general quality of care, waiting time, and the experience of the doctors in the local SF's clinics. Apart from well-qualified doctors and specialists, location of its clinic, pharmacy, and affiliated hospital is the most important factor upon which Israelis base their choice of SF.

The basic benefits available to the Israelis are called "the Health Basket." What is in it is annually determined by the Ministry of Health, based on recommendations of a public committee that includes experts in health-care, economics, and so on. The Basket includes a wide variety of services: diagnosis and treatment for adults, pregnant women (including fertility treatment) and children; hospitalization and surgeries (including transplants); prescription drugs; laboratory services (SFs have their own labs); and dental care both for adults and children (which constitutes about 9% of the health cost). Treatment of alcoholism and drug abuse is also in the Basket. Psychiatric care is covered, though visits to psychologists are not. The list of what is covered is long.[6] In 2012 the Basket was expanded, having focused on preventive care: preventive checkup, pre-natal care, dental and psychiatric care. Among the newly approved services are: vaccinations against the papilloma virus linked to cervical cancer (available to 52,000 teenage girls); genetic tests for couples planning pregnancy (some 143,000 Israelis are annually eligible); ultrasound test that checks pregnant women for certain fetal birth defects (affecting some 52,000 women). Eighty-eight innovating drugs and technologies are also added to the Basket.

Not included in the Basket are private services (lab tests, nurses, private ambulances, etc.), complementary medicine. Unfortunately, this list is also long.

Medical care in Israel is provided on three levels. What is not covered through the Health Basket can be partly picked up by a supplemental insurance, which is purchased through one's SF. About 75% of Israelis do that. SFs offer supplemental insurance on two or three levels for an additional fee, which is the same for all SFs. Such insurance enables a patient to choose his/her own doctor (rather than the doctor assigned by the SF), as well as to see doctors (and be operated on) in private clinics and hospitals; it can also slash the waiting time for hospitalization. Some prescription drugs that are not in the Basket can be purchased at a discount.

The third level is a supplemental *private* insurance. Private insurances are not regulated and work very much like in America: they may reject an applicant because of pre-existing conditions or manipulate premiums according to their "risk." However, private insurance covers many "extras": staying in a private hospital, cosmetic surgery, enhanced long-term care, and other benefits outside the Health Basket[4] If the private insurance pays for anything that could have been covered by the SF's supplemental insurance, the SF partly or completely reimburses the patient. About a third of Israelis have some comprehensive private insurance policy or private long-term care insurance. Private insurance is an alternative for those who are sick and tired of SF's bureaucracy. Not only it helps in major issues, it can help in "little things" like getting one's appointment in two days rather than two months.

Although one can see his/her family doctor or pediatrician the same day, the waiting time for a specialist appointment or a test may be quite long: according to one source, the wait is up to two weeks for a gynecologist or an ultrasound appointment. However, I learned from an Israeli friend that one could wait for a specialist appointment for up to three months. The waiting time to see a specialist also depends on where the patient lives: it may be up to six weeks in the country's north or south, whereas in the center it may be half that time. How much one waits depends on one's SF and even on one's age. Supplemental and private insurances do slash those times.

Low-income citizens, both Arab and Jewish, as well as the elderly, often cannot afford private insurance, which significantly supplements the Health Basket. Moreover, when people of that category are sick, they often hesitate to see doctors for fear that if they are diagnosed with a serious illness, they will be unable to pay for the treatment. And yet, "Myers-JDC-Brookdale Institute consistently shows 88 percent of Israelis report a high level of satisfaction with their health plans. Notably, that figure is even higher among minorities: The percentage of respondents who were satisfied or very satisfied was highest among Arabic-speaking, at 94 percent."[7]*

Israeli health care is financed through three sources: health tax withheld through payroll (which covers only 25% of health-care costs), subsidies by Bituach Leumi (BL) – the government's Israeli Insurance Institute (the equivalent of the American Social Security Administration), and directly by the government. The BL (health) tax is progressive: one pays 3.1% from earnings that is half the average wage ($2,500 as of Feb. 2011), and 4.8% from the rest of earnings up to 5 times the average wage. The self-employed pay the same taxes. As of 1996, employers do not contribute to the health tax although they do contribute to the so-called social security tax. Old age pensioners pay 2% of their average income. Housewives and working teenagers under the age 18 do not pay the tax. If both spouses work, they pay the tax separately.[8]

The health taxes withheld from payroll are transferred to BL, which distributes the funds among the SFs and also partly subsidizes them from its own funds. Government subsidies are distributed among the SFs according to the number of enrollees, the subsidies for the elderly being higher than those for younger people (e.g., 75% of the elderly are enrolled in the Clalit; therefore its government subsidy is significantly higher). Doctors and hospitals are directly reimbursed by SFs. Even if patients do not pay health insurance dues, their SFs may not refuse to pay for treatments.

The health tax, like American FICA, has a ceiling. Parts of incomes that are higher than five times the average earnings are exempted from the health tax. This is a matter of argument and confrontation among political parties, but the prevailing opinion is "if it works, don't touch!"

Israel has 264 hospitals: 48 general hospitals, 25 psychiatric clinics, 184 chronic-care hospitals, 2 rehabilitation clinics, and 5 maternity hospitals. Some hospitals belong to SFs (Clalit owns 19 hospitals!), some to the government, some are affiliated with universities, and some are private. The non-SF hospitals accept SFs' payments (with possible co-pays). There are just a few strictly private hospitals, which charge the patient their own fees (a SF and a private insurance may pick up that cost).

Some Israeli hospitals – such as Shaare Zedek, Soroka or Hadassah – are world-famous. All Israeli hospitals, with only a few exceptions, provide high-quality care.

---

* Arab Israelis give such high approval probably because they can favorably compare the services they enjoy with those outside "the Green Line" – in the area of Palestinian Autonomy.

Who Cares about Health Care?

Belonging to a SF makes an Israeli feel secure. Together with the SF's supplemental insurance, issues not requiring serious intervention are easily resolved. If the issue is serious, the patient is referred by the SF to a hospital, possibly one belonging to the SF. The patient may request referral to a different hospital.

On average, an Israeli stays in a hospital for 4 days. Some tests or procedures may be performed in outpatient departments or day clinics. Israeli health care focuses on out-of hospital treatment, the main load being placed on family doctors. Ninety percent of Israelis have regular contact with their PCPs, who are also the gatekeepers to all other medical services.

Today Israel has 3.3 doctors per 1000 population (we have only 2.5!) – which is a lot – and yet the hospitals feel the shortage of doctors. There are not enough specialty doctors, although their number is three times larger than that of PCPs. The immigration of Soviet Jews in the 1990s doubled the number of doctors, but now that many doctors are retiring, in some 20 years there will be a serious shortage of physicians.

One of the causes of the scarcity of doctors is that only about 400 new doctors join the medical force annually. Israel has five medical schools, which are all affiliated with major universities.

Interest in the medical profession has always been high in Israel. In spite of the fact that a doctor does not make much money, Israelis regard humanity highly: *every life is precious* ("Whoever saves a life, it is as if he saved an entire world" – the Talmud). Hence the desire of many young people to devote their lives to medicine. This desire is definitely influenced by the fact that most of Israel's young people have to serve in the Israeli Defense Force (IDF) after graduating from high school: boys for three years and girls for two.* Only after their army service can they enter a university. Their military experience enhances for them the value of human life.

In order to be accepted to a medical school one does not need a bachelor's degree. A high school diploma is sufficient. Upon returning from the army, the youngsters typically spend a year traveling or working to earn money to pay for their education. Sometimes a year of remedial study is necessary. Thus, an Israeli young man or woman is ready for a university or a medical school at age 23 or 24 and graduates at 30.

The competition to be accepted to a medical school is intense. In 2011, out of

---

* The most brilliant young people may be granted postponement of their military service. They are allowed to enter a university or a medical school on the condition that after graduating they will be working – in their new specialty – for the IDF (typically for five years).

1,600 applicants only about 400 were accepted. Medical schools in other countries (primarily the former Soviet Union, Romania and Hungary) also train a few hundred Israelis.

In order to receive an MD diploma, one typically has to study six years and then do a year of rotating internships. In the first three years students study basic science, and focus on clinical studies in the last three. After the first three years they receive a BS degree in medical sciences.

Medical school (as well as university education) in Israel is not free. For each of the first three years tuition is approximately $2,500, whereas in the clinical years it is $3,250 (as of 2011).[9] * This fee covers 10%–13% of the cost of tuition. The rest is paid by the government in the form of grants to medical schools. "Part of the implicit social contract between the country and its young people is that, in exchange for this [army] service, the state will cover most of the costs of their higher education."[11]

An Israeli physician earns $60,000–$75,000 a year. This is significantly less than one would make in the U.S. However, against the background of generally lower salaries in Israel, a doctor earns 3 times more than the average salary (an American doctor earns 5.5 times more).

In a blog, I found the following response to a question asked by an American doctor who was contemplating immigrating to Israel.

> In Israel, to be a doctor requires you to be very smart, and thus anyone who is a doctor is well respected for their intelligence and their desire to help people even if they make a poor salary.

Nevertheless, in the afternoons, thousands of doctors rush to their second jobs at private clinics or hospitals.

As I mentioned, there may be a waiting time for hospitalization. However, in an emergency, hospitalization is immediate. *Magen David Adom* (Red Star of David) is the organization responsible for immediate response to any health emergency situations.

MDA has 700 ambulances, among them basic life support and mobile intensive care units. Some ambulances are armored: these are sent to locations of terrorist acts and respond to emergency calls from settlements outside the Green Line. Sometimes they are fired upon despite their clearly visible MDA insignias. Ambulances are based at 95 MDA stations throughout the country. The average time of waiting for an ambulance's arrival is 10 to 40 minutes, depending on location.

---

* The tuition fee for receiving a bachelor's degree at universities is also $2,500/year.

Who Cares about Health Care?

Apart from a mobile response to health emergencies, Israel has 850 first aid stations located at such places as malls, stadiums, city locations where there may be crowding, and so on. The station is simply a box with the medicine and resuscitation equipment necessary for an immediate response to a heart attack, stroke, or other emergency. Only specially trained paramedics have access to the box. The station fits into a motorcycle rack so it is easily movable, even in a mall.

MDA has approximately 1,200 paramedics, technicians and emergency doctors. Twelve thousand volunteers are an intrinsic part of MDA operations. Youngsters 15-18 years old undergo special training and then actively participate in emergency operations. There is also an international program that accepts 18-year-old volunteers.

The MDA volunteer program also has an important social function. It serves as a youth club, strengthening youngsters' social conscience. After their army service, many former volunteers return to MDA, serving in emergency situations as drivers and medics. Especially active are those who had in the army medical specialty.

Israel has another emergency services organization, completely volunteer and independent of MDA. It is called United Hatzalah (rescue)[*10]. There are over 2000 volunteers trained as paramedics who ride motorcycles ("ambucycles") equipped with first aid stations (boxes with first aid equipment, including defibrillators) and arrive at sites where first aid is required within just a few (typically three!) minutes. An ambulance, which has to fight traffic, arrives later, when the necessary first aid has been done.

This organization was created 20 years ago by Eli Beer, who is now its president. The organization is non-profit and supported only through donations. All the UH's services are free, and the volunteers are unpaid and do not accept tips. The organization is proud of being "united," with Arabs' volunteers working alongside Jews. Like MDA, the UH's volunteers work 24-7 without holidays. When a police call arrives at the organization information system, the volunteers closest to the emergency site are informed. They stop work immediately (no matter what their jobs are), jump onto their motorcycles and in three minutes begin their rescue missions. In 2013, UH saved 40,000 lives.[11]

---

[*] The very first volunteer first aid organization was created in Brooklyn, NY, by orthodox Jews to service their communities. The very simple idea that a motorbike can beat any traffic is gradually spreading outside Israel. Quite possibly, it could also be implemented in the U.S. However, in American towns and in rural areas, ambulances are mostly sent from the nearest fire stations, avoiding traffic. And most likely we will not be able to compete with Israeli's idealism.

However, although UH ambucycles save thousands of lives, it is an MDA ambulance that will bring a patient to a nearby emergency room or a specific SF hospital.* There, the treatment is similar to that of a good American hospital. But suppose one has not called 101 for an MDA ambulance and arrives at the nearest ER on one's own. (We all know what an American ER is like: even in a good hospital, one can sit in a reception room for a long time before seeing a doctor. That's why smart advice to an American is to call 911 no matter what. You will be taken directly to a doctor and avoid an ER.) As for Israel, here I want to tell my own story.

During my trip to Israel in 2010, I got sick with severe abdominal pains. My friend brought me directly to the ER at Tel HaShomer hospital in the center of Israel, east of Ramat Gan. There were some 50 or so people sitting there. Upon registration (the girl spoke perfect English), I was asked to sit. But in just 10 or so minutes I was called to a doctor's office. Within a few minutes, a young female physician compiled the "anamnesis" – the history of my present and previous sicknesses–and sent me for blood and urine tests and an X-ray. That took another 20 minutes. Then I was directed to wait at the office of another doctor. Here I lost about 20 minutes because the doctor twice mispronounced my name so that I could not recognize it. When I eventually saw him, he explained, again in good English, what the possible diagnoses might be, based on my X-ray and tests. One of them was not very good, so he suggested (actually insisted) that I stay in the hospital for further tests. I refused, saying that I had to fly home in just two days. "Try to fly tomorrow," he said. It was one day before the Passover holiday, and even if I agreed to stay, nothing would be done because most doctors would be out observing the holiday. While I stood in a short line to pay for services, a nurse came up and said that she had to give me a supply of antibiotics for two days. When it was my turn to see the cashier, I was astonished to see my bill: $261.74. I asked if it was possible to break it down so that I could see how much the different procedures cost, but the girl said no, this was the charge for the whole visit. I probably spent not more than an hour and a half in the ER. The next day I purchased some more antibiotics at a drug store. Without health insurance, it cost me $33. Two days later I returned to Boston. The "bad diagnosis" proved false and in a couple of weeks I was healthy. My insurance reimbursed me, minus the cost of antibiotics and minus $100. I had a co-pay of $100 because I had visited an ER. (Isn't that funny? No –absurd! A person gets penalized for having an urgent health problem!)

This was my experience with an Israeli ER. Researching through the Internet, I came across other confirmations of my experience, especially in blogs where

---

*If the patient is not hospitalized, he/she has to pay the ambulance bill.

people shared their opinions.

I have been unable to find out how much an Israeli doctor pays as a malpractice insurance premium. A doctor I asked answered that she did not know how much she paid because the premium was deducted from her salary. One source insisted that the malpractice insurance in Israel is much less expensive than in the U.S. On the other hand, lawyers do collect contingency fees in litigations – a plague in the U.S.

Maternity.[12] In Israel, a pregnant woman has a 14-week maternity leave, which she can split as she likes. After she has given birth she is automatically eligible for another 12 weeks of unpaid leave, which can be extended to 26 weeks. The pregnant woman's SF takes care of her during pregnancy (consultations, check-ups, ultra-sound) and after giving birth.

During the 14-week leave a working, woman receives reimbursement of her salary from BL, rather than from her SF. The check is issued after delivery, rather than when the paid leave begins. (The universal principle: if one must pay, pay as late as possible!)

Women must give birth in a hospital (or arrive there immediately after) or else the delivery will not be covered. The delivery is attended by a midwife or nurse unless a doctor's presence is necessary. The woman may have a doctor present at delivery if she is staying in a private hospital or has private insurance accepted by the public hospital.

The cost of delivery and stay in a hospital is paid by BL in the form of a grant directly to the hospital. The grant also covers the cost of hospitalizing the baby should it be necessary. A BL's special grant covers the parents' expenses: about $470 for the first child and roughly $3,500 for the birth of triplets.

The child has his/her own Health Basket:

> The "Basket of Child Development Services" provides child development care for children up to the age of 9 (in some cases up to age 18). Included are diagnosis and treatment by multi-disciplinary teams for children with speech and language disorders and impediments, minor neurological dysfunctions, certain somatic disorders, attention deficit disorders, and learning disabilities. For some types of treatments, parents are required to cover some of the costs, depending on the child's age and other factors. Specific inoculations are given routinely at fixed intervals throughout the baby's first years, including polio, diphtheria, whooping cough, tetanus, and measles.[13]

A high percentage of Israeli women work outside the home. After the 14-week paid leave is over, most women take additional unpaid leave. After that the family has to find day care for their child.

There are a few options.[14] Apart from babysitters and other private arrangements, parents can send their child to a state or private kindergarten. The private kindergartens accept children from 3 months to 5 years. They are supervised by the Ministry of Education. The public kindergartens are for children from 3 to 6 years old; they are subdivided into three age groups: 3-4, 4-5, and 5-6. The staff of the government–run kindergartens is usually well trained and experienced. There, the children get a good pre-school education. Five-to-six-year-old children may enter a primary school (schooling is mandatory from grades 5 through grades 10 or 12). If a child is not ready for primary school intellectually or psychologically, he/she stays in kindergarten for another year.

Now I jump from the very young to the very old.

Long-term health care (LTC) insurance.[15] Like everywhere in developed countries, the Israeli population is aging. Israel has one of the highest life expectancies at birth in the world – 81.7 years (women –83.6, men –79.9). Therefore the percentage of the population 65 and older is growing dramatically: * in 2014 it was 10.3%, and is expected to be 14% in 2030. Moreover, almost half of that group was comprised of the elderly, 75 and older. Seventy percent of the elderly who need in-house assistance are women. Since 1988, LTC insurance is a part of the National Health Insurance Law.

> The [Law] covers disabled men aged 67 and over and disabled women of 62 years of age and over who are permanent residents of Israel. It also covers new immigrants who arrived in Israel after reaching retirement age. Eligibility is subject to an income test. Its upper limits are 1.5 times and 2.25 times the average wage for individuals and couples, respectively, thus excluding only 1.3% of applicants from benefit entitlement.[13]

Eligible people undergo assessments and may be eligible for 10, 16 or 18 hours of care per week, depending on how many basic functions (out of 6 internationally accepted "Activities of Daily Living" [ADL]), they cannot fulfill. Failure to fulfill 3 basic functions makes a patient eligible for LTC insurance (dementia and Alzheimer's disease also count). The helpers oversee

---

* "Statistically, if you reach the age of 65 in Israel, and you stand an excellent chance of doing so, then you have a 1 in 3 chance of needing long-term nursing care before you reach 120" (a Q&A blog). (In the Jewish tradition, based on the Bible, 120 is the maximal age a human being is allowed. Hence a toast – "may you live to 120!").

the elderly, help around the house with hygiene, do grocery shopping, laundry, and so on. They are rarely paid in cash.

"Generic" LTC care is financed by both the insured and the government. As of 2011, all Israelis pay a special tax of 0.14% of their wages (collected by BL), and employers contribute another 0.09% for a total of 0.23%. The government (through BL) contributes another 0.02% of the insured's wage.

Home care is expensive; the cost can be as high as $3,000 a month. All four SFs offer their members additional group policies. They provide some extra coverage for around $1,300 a month for three years, and $700 for another two years. The money is paid only as a reimbursement for expenses. Private insurance companies also offer policies: one can purchase various types of coverage (up to $6,000/month) and for various periods of time. Private funding comprises close to 50% of LTC expenses.

A nursing home stay is quite expensive: private nursing home costs can be over $6,000/month (in the U.S. it is at least $9,000). Government nursing homes, which are less expensive, have waiting lists.

The LTC care system in Israel has a very complex structure. There is a network of assisted living complexes of various levels of care and cost. One source suggested that a patient contemplating moving to one of the available facilities should consult a lawyer.

No matter how much support a family can purchase, there is also family caregiving mostly by members of the elderly person's family. Israel has a strong tradition of caring for parents, grandparents and other family members.

How healthy are Israelis? The leading causes of death in Israel are the same as in all developed countries: two thirds of deaths are caused by heart disease, cancer, and stroke. Israelis eat too much: 28.0% of women and 40.7% of men are overweight; 14.9%/17.1% of women/men are obese (see table in Conclusion); 16% of 20-64 year-olds have high cholesterol.

No matter what the country, health status has been found to correlate with the socioeconomic condition of its people. The health status of low-income Arab citizens and Jews is lower than that of affluent Israelis. The life expectancy of low-income Arabs is 3.7 years lower than that of Jews, mostly because of the difference in lifestyle, including poor hygiene, more smoking, and less exercise. Childhood mortality among low-income Arab citizens, Mizrahi Jews (originating from the Middle East, Africa and the Caucasus), and Ethiopian immigrants is higher than among Ashkenazi (European and American) Jews. The mortality rate also depends on geographic location: how far away or how accessible the nearest SF facility is.

The health care of Arab Israelis has been at the center of left-right bickering for years. Arab Israelis, like all Israeli citizens, have to belong to one of the four SFs. Their benefits are exactly the same. After the National Health-Care Law was passed in 1995, a network of clinics was built in the areas with a high Arab population. Many doctors and nurses are Arabs who graduated from Israeli medical or other schools. (The Hadassah Medical Center – one of the world's highest acclaimed – is famous for training Arab medical personnel.) Much has been done to improve medical services to the Arab population. In spite of these advances, an enormous number of lies have been spread by the international media about Israel's "racism" and "atrocities." This is sad. It is especially sad that too often it is the Israeli left that disseminates those lies.

Israel is often accused of failing to "exercise responsibility" for Palestinians' health care. However, a few years ago Israel offered the Palestinian Authority $11 million worth of medicine, but the Palestinians turned down the offer, requesting cash instead. That was not the only suggestion aimed at cooperation.

An Aid Equipment Lending Center functions in Ramalla, a joint project of Israel's Joint Distribution Committee and the Palestinian Medical Relief Committees. Rear Admiral Dr. Susan Blumenthal, former U.S. Assistant Surgeon General, heads the Palestinian/Israeli Health Initiative (supported by a grant from USAID).[16]

In 2012, according to Civil Administration annual summary, approximately 220,000 Palestinian patients (among them 21,000 children) were treated in Israeli hospitals, over 100 Palestinian doctors interned at Israeli hospitals, and more than five organ donations were performed."[17]

As for day-to-day medical help for Palestinians, in January 2011, CNN aired the story of the fight for life of Aya Abu Mouwais, a 3-year-old Palestinian girl.[18] Yuval Roth, a carpenter, founded the organization "On the Road to Recovery." Together with 200 volunteers, Roth provides transportation of sick people from the West Bank to Israeli hospitals. In the past two years, little Aya and her mother were driven 200 times to Rambam Medical Center, where the necessary treatment was administered.

This is not an isolated case of medical help to Palestinians. Regretfully, there have been situations (fortunately not many) when Palestinians whose lives were saved in Israeli hospitals later attempted to commit suicide bombings.[*]

---

[*] In 2011 the Israeli documentary *Precious Life* was nominated for an Oscar. The film is about a Gaza woman whose son was born without immune system and would die without a bone marrow transplant that could only be performed in an Israeli hospital. The fund-raising among Israelis raised the necessary money to pay for the

Who Cares about Health Care?

As I mentioned, Israel has first-class medical facilities. They attract what is called "medical tourism." – traveling to Israel to receive medical treatment.[19] *
Approximately 15,000 foreigners come to Israel annually for treatment (35% of them for cosmetic surgeries). Many procedures here are up to 50% less expensive than in the UK or America. For example, heart replacement is just $20,000 to 35,000 vs. $125,000 in America. Cosmetic surgery is just around 20% cheaper: a facelift costs $7,000 compared to $8,500 in America.[17]

Israel also has advanced procedures and effective experimental drugs for treating cancer. For many cancer patients, Israel is the last resort and hope.

What can I say in conclusion? Israel is the country I love. I tried to be objective and not conceal her faults. Among them is a huge bureaucracy that makes almost any step in receiving good health care difficult. Endless forms must be filled out; endless referrals must be obtained.

The Israeli health-care system is often accused of being socialistic. However, it is neither a completely government directed nor a single-payer system. Israel was founded as a socialist state. Until the end of the 1970s, there was virtually no economic entity that was not controlled by the government. Since then, especially after the privatization drive initiated by Benjamin Netanyahu's activity from 1996 as Israeli Finance- and Prime minister, a lot has changed in Israel, including its health-care system. And yet, some socialist features do remain. There is competition among SFs, in which the government does not interfere, although each SF is a tightly self-controlled system. Fortunately, there are ways to escape that system through private insurance that at least one-third of Israelis purchase.

To an average Israeli, health-care expenses are not too heavy a burden. The government gives subsidies to poor people that help them make ends meet. As I mentioned, Israelis are highly satisfied with their system.

Health-care expenses consume 8% of Israel's GDP – on par with other European countries, but half of the U.S.' expenses. Like the health-care systems in the other countries we visited, the Israeli system is approaching a crisis of "invasion" of the elderly. In the near future Israel will experience a shortage of doctors. To help offset this shortage, the organization Nefesh

---

surgery (an Israeli who had lost his son in a war donated $55,000). After the successful surgery, the boy's mother said that she had wanted to save her son's life so that in the future he would become a shahid. She later changed her mind. A sad story.   (http://www.foxnews.com/entertainment/2011/01/13/precious-life-suicide-bomber-shlomi-edar/).

* In 2010, an Arab princess (daughter of a royal family in the Persian Gulf), chose to have life-saving heart surgery in Israel (http://www.israelnationalnews.com/News/News.aspx/140778#).

Israel

B'Nefesh (Jewish Souls United)[20] offers physicians who would like to immigrate to Israel significant benefits.

Israel may also expect a massive immigration of Jews from Europe, where anti-Semitism is rampant. Immigration also rises with the increasing political power of the Muslims. Without a radical change in the health-care system, more government subsidies will be needed. The ability of the government to increase its support will, of course, depend on the overall economic situation in Israel.

The current world economic crisis has not affected Israel as much as other countries, and recovery was much faster. The quick economic recovery and high growth rate (4.8% in 2011) are mostly due to Israel's concentration on biomedical technology and high-tech industries. As I mentioned, Israel has more start-up companies per capita than any other country, and may become a high-tech super-power within the nearest decade. One of the break-throughs that may be expected is development of a substitute for oil (while solar and wind energy are still in cradles). Huge funds for this purpose have been provided by major world investors. Huge deposits of natural gas have been recently discovered and Israel began exporting liquefied gas to Europe, which dramatically changes the Europe's economy.

Let me complete this visit to Israel with the hope that Israel will emerge strengthened from today's calamities and that its health-care system will survive and flourish.

3. OBAMACARE:
Patient Protection and Affordable Care Act

"We need change! Yes, we can!"
Barak Obama' 2008 election
campaign slogan

The *Patient Protection and Affordable Care Act*[*,1,2,3] was passed by the House on March 21, 2010, and signed into law by President Obama on March 23. A health care reform was long overdue, and Americans were waiting for it. However, the polls showed that the majority of Americans (56%) did not support the overall legislation, although some provisions were broadly supported. After the 2010 midterm election just a few months after the bill was passed, the new Republican majority in the House immediately began to assault the bill. In January 2011, the Republican House voted to repeal it. However, with president's veto in store, the repeal of the bill in the near future seems impossible.

The constitutionality of the ACA has also been challenged. Twenty-eight states, as well as many organizations and individuals, have launched lawsuits against the bill. The Supreme Court's hearing took place on March 26-28, 2012. In its June 28th ruling, the Court upheld the ACA, albeit with some reservations.[4]

Right after the bill was passed, e-mails of millions of people became clogged with messages containing a lot of false information emanating both from the left and the right. Being among those millions, I decided not to forward them until I learned more about the plan.

Since the passage of the bill over four years ago, the "fog of the controversy" that Nancy Pelosi wanted to look through[†] not only had thinned but even thickened. However, after the Supreme Court decisions and numerous comments on it, the situation begins to emerge a bit more clearly. Books have been published on the subject. If you type "Obamacare" into the Amazon.com book section, you will see over 1000 entries, and they are multiplying! And

---

[*] Usually abbreviated as PPACA; I will be using ACA.
[†] N. Pelosi: "We have to pass the bill so that you can find out what is in it away from the fog of the controversy": http://www.youtube.com/watch?v=hV-05TLiiLU.

yet, the April 2013 Kaiser Family Foundation poll[5] revealed that "about half the public says they do not have enough information about the health reform law to understand how it will impact their own family."

After the malfunction of the government website that was supposed to allow people to enroll in Obamacare, and the explosion of the controversy over President Obama's retraction from his earlier claim: "if you like your health care plan, you can keep your health care plan," the fog thickened some more. Partly because of controversial and sometimes contradictory claims by Obamacare supporters, many still do not understand how their health care will look after 2014. As of February 2014, not all people who believe they should enroll in Obamacare were able to do so because of software malfunction. But the main problem is ahead, when people will begin comparing their former bills with the anticipated ones, and discover that the doctor they would like to see is unavailable. Also, those who intend to purchase insurance through their employers still do not know what kind of policies they will have and how much they will pay for them. There is a danger that many people will decide not to enroll to Obamacare, rather agreeing to pay penalties ("taxes").

Therefore, I am in an ambivalent position. On the one hand, the situation with Obamacare is still too volatile. Possibly no one is able to predict what Obamacare will look like in 2016. On the other hand, I have spent a lot of time attempting to understand the ACA, and would like to share with my readers what I learned. Besides, without some information about the future of American health care this book would have been lame, especially, after we have seen from the previous chapter how health care systems are organized and function in other countries.

In investigating the new bill, I have attempted to be as objective as possible, which means that too often I was in "no man's land." To sift through GOOGLE entries on the ACA was not an easy task. Apart from rejecting false information, one must carefully discriminate between the ACA Bill H.R. 3962 of 2009, the final bill of the same number entitled *Preservation of Access to Care for Medicare Beneficiaries and Pension Relief Act of 2010* signed by President Obama into law on June 25, 2010, and *H.R. 4872. Health Care and Education Reconciliation Act of 2010*. The final bill has quite a few important amendments that eliminate some controversial or politically unacceptable clauses. And changes are still coming.

Here are the sources I borrowed from most often: The complete bill; the government website (mostly questions and answers)[6]; the ObamaCare Facts site,[7] (containing links to different aspects of the reform); the Kaiser Family Foundation (one of the most reliable source, periodically updating its information)[8]; National Federation of Independent Businesses (a very detailed information source);[9] the RAND Corporation[10]; the Cato Institute[11]; the Congressional Budget Office[12] and others.

While I was writing this chapter, the book *Inside National Health Care* by John E. McDough, one of the architects of the ACA reform, was published (University of California Press, Berkeley, 2011). An overview of the book can be found in Medscape.com's *What's Really in the Affordable Care Act*.[13]

To begin with, why did we need health care reform?

The main reason for changes – and virtually all agree – is the huge number of uninsured Americans. How many are they?

Prior to the ACA, the numbers of uninsured were reported to vary from 46 to 66 million. The 2012 U.S. Census Bureau document[14] gave the number of uninsured in 2011 as 48.6 million.* The Congressional Budget Office (CBO) estimates[12] the number of uninsured in 2012 as 53 million. When collecting data, the Census Bureau uses independent estimates of population (the so-called "population control" technique); therefore the number of uninsured that it posts is quite reliable. I will be using that number because the CBO estimate includes "unauthorized immigrants."

Quite a few conservative sources claim that the actual number is significantly smaller (up to only 6-8 million);[15] Among the alleged mistaken counting are 9.3 million uninsured legal residents who are not citizens, 8.9 million uninsured young people age 18-24 (they just do not want to be insured!), as well as "affluent people" who for some reasons have decided not to purchase health insurance: 10.6 million with incomes $50,000–$75,000 and over.

Unauthorized immigrants definitely should not be counted among the uninsured. However, should we exclude all legal non-citizens? This would be wrong because they work and pay taxes. The only difference between these people and citizens is that they do not vote, but 50% of eligible citizens do not vote either.

Why "affluent" people do not wish to purchase insurance is anyone's guess. However, with an average cost of insurance for a family being $15,000/year[16], even those who earn $50,000 can hardly afford to pay over one third of their income after taxes for insurance.

Some low-income people may be eligible for government subsistence (Medicaid), but have not enrolled. However, it is again anyone's guess how

---

* According to the Census Bureau, the "uninsured" are people who were not covered by any health insurance for the entire year.

many of them should be removed from the total number of uninsured.

We definitely should not remove uninsured young people. Some of them do not want to purchase insurance because they naively believe that nothing can happen to them. However, many young adults working for companies that do not provide health insurance simply cannot afford to purchase it. We will see that Obamacare will take care of this category of the uninsured.

Actually, the discussion of those conservative numbers does not make sense. The Census Bureau data give a detailed picture of who the uninsured are. From the document I have already referenced,[14] one can see that among the 48.6 million uninsured there are 7.6 million children under the age of 19; 8.3 million young people age 19-26, at least 23 million adults slightly above the poverty level, and over 10 million "uninsurable" with some pre-existing conditions.

Thus, let us stick with the Census Bureau figure of 48.6 million uninsured.

Hence, *No Uninsured Left Behind* was the main goal of the reform. At least three other objectives for launching a new health care reform were:

> – Stop insurance companies from discriminating practices that refuse coverage to people with pre-existing conditions and discriminating against women.
> – Bring down the cost of health insurance by slashing bureaucracy.
> – Eliminate fraud and abuse.

Unfortunately, as estimates by RAND[10] and CBO[12] show, the main objective of the reform will not be achieved. By 2016, the number of uninsured will be slashed only to 25–26 million; by 2021 it will climb to 27 million.

The ACA law is composed of 10 Titles dealing with various aspects of the reform.[13]

Title I. Quality, Affordable Health Care for All Americans: a new system of purchasing health insurance (Exchanges).
Title II. The Role of Public Programs: establishes significant changes to Medicaid.
Title III. Improving the Quality and Efficiency of Health Care: "establishes new mechanisms to improve the quality of medical care in the United States by making it more efficient and effective, and more patient-centered."
Title IV. Prevention of Chronic Disease and the Improvement of Public Health: establishes a National Prevention, Health Promotion, and Public Health Council.
Title V. Health Care Workforce: establishes a National Health Care Workforce Commission to plan workforce needs and expansion.

Title VI. Transparency and Program Integrity: focuses on combating fraud and abuse in the system. It also establishes the Patient Centered Outcomes Research Institute "to support research on comparative clinical effectiveness."

Title VII. Improving Access to Innovative Medical Therapies: supports development and use of generic drugs.

Title VIII. CLASS: Community Living Assistance Supports and Services: long-term disability program, later repealed.

Title IX. Revenue Provisions: covers new Medicare and other taxes and surcharges, providing half of the necessary financing.

Title X. Strengthening Quality, Affordable Health Care for All Americans: includes amendments and additions to Titles I-IX, approved by separate legislation (HCERA).

It is relatively easy to understand what Titles I and II mean. I will focus mostly on them. Other Titles are rather foggy, and I will only be touching on what I understand there.

Before going to the first reform objective, let me first in just a few words review the health insurance situation in America before ACA.[7]

As we already agreed upon, about 15% of our population ($48.6 million) were uninsured. What about the others? Insured through employers: 48%; insured by Medicaid: 15% and Medicare: 5%; "non-group" (those who purchased their policies on the free market): 5%, and those under government health care: 2%. Thus, 85% of the population had health insurance. It is obvious that, in order to insure the millions of uninsured, the government had to find ways to pay for it. I will be discussing this issue below. This is a hot spot, because many people will have to pay more than before (even significantly more) for their health care, which may be a source of political complications.

Let me now begin with the first objective:

No Uninsured Left Behind.

Ideally, the first objective could be achieved if health insurance were mandatory. That is what the individual mandate is all about: the requirement that most U. S. citizens and legal residents purchase at least "minimum coverage" (determined by government) either through an employer or individually through an insurance market.

This is the individual mandate that has been the main accusation of unconstitutionality directed against Obamacare: one cannot force anyone to purchase no matter what, if one does not want it. This should also apply to health insurance as a commodity. However, the Supreme Court has upheld the constitutionality of the individual mandate clause.

In a nutshell, this is how the individual mandate will work.

–Everyone must be covered by an insurance plan either through employers or through individual purchase on the insurance market.

(Transition to the new law would be easier if [as people have been assured] one who already had a good insurance policy would be able to keep it. Unfortunately, President Obama's claim that those who had insurance before might keep it was not supported by the ACA law. Actually, in order to be "grandfathered," health plans had to be operational before March 23, 2010, that is, before the ACA was signed into law. In order to save the grandfathering privileges, employers could slightly tinker with the plans they had been offering earlier. All plans have to agree with government Essential Health Benefits.)

–An insured may add to his/her policy a spouse or children up to the age of 26. However, some employers who offered a health plan before the ACA may refuse to do it now, even under the threat of fines.

–All health care or gender discriminations will be prohibited.

Now the details:

Beginning in 2015, those failing to be insured will pay a phased-in tax penalty,[*] reaching 1%, 2% and 2.5% of taxable income respectively in 2014, 2015 and 2016. In 2016, a family that refused to join the system will have to pay a maximum penalty of $2,085.[17] Those earning less than an income threshold will be exempted from paying a penalty and thus will be allowed to remain uninsured. And yet, according to the CBO[18] about 7 million Americans will have to pay penalties averaging about $1,000. By 2021 this will bring the government some $45 billion.[12]

A new online insurance market, the American Health Benefit Exchanges, has been created, through which individuals will be able to purchase coverage. As for mid-2014, only 16 states (plus DC) had their own Exchanges. Separate Small Business Health Options Program (SHOP) Exchanges will also be created for each state, through which employers of up to 100 employees will be obligated to purchase insurance policies for their employees.

Buying health insurance online was presumed to be as easy as buying online car insurance. Upon entering the Exchange page, prospective buyers would have to fill out a questionnaire, which includes a request for their income.

––––––––––––––––––––

[*] In order to collect the penalty taxes, the IRS will have to hire close to 12,000 new agents.

After that they will be presented with possible choices: Medicaid, CHIP, * or buying a standardized health plan.

A state may organize its own Exchange, or agree to have its Exchange run by a federal bureaucracy. A few states may combine their Exchanges, thus widening the Exchange market. Insurance companies participating in an Exchange will be competing for buyers. By mid-2014 the Exchange system was hoped to have been operational.

As I mentioned, the ACA requires all health insurance plans either sold by businesses or purchased individually through Exchanges, to provide Essential Health Benefits, a minimum package of services. The package must include services within the following ten categories:[19]

- •Ambulatory patient services
- •Emergency services
- •Hospitalization
- •Maternity and newborn care
- •Mental health and substance use disorder services, including behavioral health treatment
- •Prescription drugs
- •Rehabilitative and habilitative services and devices
- •Laboratory services
- •Preventive and wellness services and chronic disease management
- •Pediatric services, including oral and vision care

This is a kind of health basket. What is covered in each of these ten categories of services is to be determined by the Secretary of Health and Human Services. Although the categories are ironclad, even with HHS Secretary recommendations, some insurance plans may sell slightly different options or may not sell some of them. Among the options are different out-of-pocket policy costs: deductibles, co-payments and drug coverage. This health basket is different, for example, from those, say, in France or Israel: there, what is covered is precisely formulated and nothing can be excluded.

The Essential Health Benefits will be available in four categories:[8]

---

* The Children's Health Insurance Program, administered by Balanced Budget Act of 1997, is "the largest expansion of taxpayer-funded health insurance coverage for children in the U.S. since Medicaid began in the 1960s." It "provides matching funds to states for health insurance to families with children. The program was designed with the intent to cover uninsured children in families with incomes that are modest but too high to qualify for Medicaid." (http://en.wikipedia.org/wiki/ State_Children %27s_Health_Insurance_Program).

OBAMACARE

•The Bronze plan represents minimum creditable coverage and provides essential health benefits. Its premiums would cover 60% of the benefit costs of the plan;
•The Silver plan covers 70% of the benefit costs of the plan;
•The Gold plan covers 80% of the benefit costs of the plan;
•The Platinum plan covers 90% of the benefit costs of the plan.

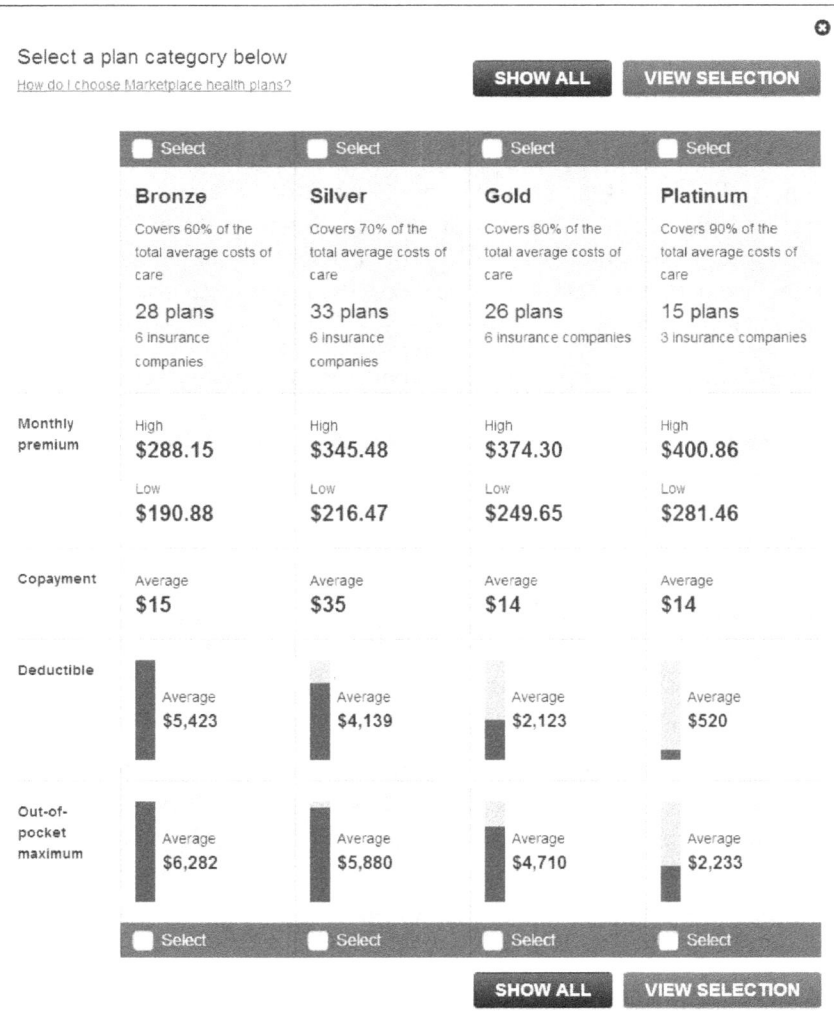

There is also a catastrophic plan available to those up to the age of 30 or to those who are exempt from the mandate to purchase insurance. This plan is only available in the individual market.

Those who are not employed or are self-employed (the so-called "non-group," some 15 million people before ACA) will have to purchase their insurance through Exchanges.

Above are the insurance options a Florida exchange offered to my friend. She had only to push the "Select" and the "View Selection" buttons and make a final decision. However, having done the arithmetic, she decided rather to pay a penalty (at least for the time being).

The key element that enabled Obamacare to extend coverage to millions of individuals and families is government subsidies. Apart from expanding Medicaid, which will pay virtually all health care costs, two kinds of subsidies are available. The first is tax credits in premium costs. They are refundable and advanceable: if the credit is larger than one's tax liability, the difference will be returned to the person, and that will be done when the payments were made (not at the time of tax return). The second is subsidies for out-of-pocket expenses.

Tax credits will be available for low-income people with incomes of up to 400% of the Federal Poverty Level (FPL). In 2013, the FPL for families of one, two, three and four was respectively $11,670, $15,130, $19,090, and $23,050. The FPL is periodically adjusted for inflation.

The Silver plan is used as a benchmark for calculating credits.

One will have to pay a definite percentage of one's income, increasing from 2% to 9.5% with income increasing from 138% to 400%FPL. The tax credit will be calculated as a difference between the Silver plan premium and that amount. If one purchases a Bronze plan, which is less expensive than the Silver plan's tax credit, the credit is not allowed.

If a family of four with an income of $46,100 (200%FLP) purchases a Silver plan, which would   cost (for example) about $8,500, the family must pay $2,904 up front – 6.3% of its income. Then it will be eligible for a tax credit of $5,596 ($8,500 minus $2,904).[20] A family with twice that income: $92,200 (400%FPL) would have to pay 9.5% of its income: $8,759, which is more than the plan cost.[*] So, they would pay the total amount of 8,500 without a credit. If

---

[*] Of course, the amount of credits depends on the plan cost. The example above uses "average" costs; see http://kff.org/interactive/subsidy-calculator/ #state= &zip=&income-type=dollars&income=46%2C100&employer-coverage=0&people=1&alternate-plan-family=individual&adult-count=2&adults%5B0%5D%5Bage%5D=21&adults%5B0%5D%5Btobacco%5D=0 &adults%5B1%5D%5Bage%5D=21&adults%5B1%5D%5Btobacco%5D=0&child-count=2&child-tobacco=0.

the family would like to purchase a Gold or Platinum plan, the tax credits would be exactly the same as for a Silver plan, $5,596 and $0.

A single with the income of $23,340 (200%FPL) would have to pay upfront $1,470 (6.3%), and the tax credit, with the cost of a Silver plan of $3,900, would be $2,430. For the income of $35,010 (300%FPL) the upfront payment would be $3,325 (9.5%), and the tax credit would be only $575. For higher incomes, tax credit would be $0.

The higher tier plans will be more expensive and may cost the same family as much as 12% of its income. High-end, the so-called Cadillac plans (with premiums at or above $10,200 for a single or $27,500 for a family) may be subject to a 40% excise tax, depending on cost.

I described these subsidies in detail because it is mostly this group of low-income people with incomes above 100%FPL that were uninsured before, and now, because of government subsidies, becomes insured. Most of these people will have to purchase their health insurance through Exchanges.

Almost all Exchange plans will have deductibles (not less than $1,250 for a single and $2,500 for a family), and co-payments for doctor visits and drugs. Those "out-of-pocket" expenses are capped at $6,250 for an individual and $12,500 for a family. They may be paid for with before-tax money from one's Health Savings Accounts.* However, most likely, HSA's money will not be enough: HSA's limits in 2013 were $3,250 for individuals and $6,450 for families.

Out-of-pocket expenses may also be subsidized for those with an income up to 250%FPL who purchase a Silver plan from their Exchange. The subsidies will cover 94% of expenses for the lowest income people and 73% for individuals and families at 250%FPL.

I apologize for so many numbers. But, as we can see, one who purchases an insurance policy through Exchanges would pay for a policy from 3% of one's income (at 138%FPL) up to about 12% for higher incomes, plus out-of-pocket expenses. If this were a health care tax, wouldn't we be angry?

Employers do not have to provide health insurance for their employees. If

---

* HSAs should not be confused with Flexible Spending Accounts (FSA), which can be opened by employees in order to pay for most health-care expenses with before-tax dollars. From 2011, payments for over-the-counter medications from FSAs are allowed only if doctors' prescriptions have been issued. Beginning with 2013, pre-tax employee contributions to FSAs were limited to $2,500/year.

they do not, and they have more than 50 employees, they will have to pay penalties. In general, employers will have to deal with a complex system of credits and penalties, depending on the number of employees and their wages. According to CBO estimates, from 2012 through 2021, businesses will pay $96 billion in penalties if they fail to provide their employees with affordable coverage.[12] Actually, in some cases, it would be cheaper for an employer to pay penalties than to provide the employees with health insurance. Then the employees will be on their own. Some 10 to 12 million people will have lost their employer's coverage; 8 to 9 million of them will end up enrolling in Medicaid,[*] thus increasing the number of enrollees by almost 25% (in 2012 the total number of Medicaid and CHIP beneficiaries was about 55 million). Others will purchase government subsidized insurances through Exchanges.[†]

Apart from this four-tier benefit system, the states will be required to create Basic Health Plans providing, as a minimum, essential health benefits (like a Bronze plan) to be offered to the uninsured with an income of 138% to 200%FPL (ineligible for Medicaid), who otherwise would have to be eligible for subsidies through Exchanges.

Within each Exchange, at least one plan has to be offered by a non-profit insurance company. As a matter of long-term policy, the Consumer Operated and Oriented Plan (CO-OP) program will be initiated, which will have to sponsor "non-profit, member-run" health insurance companies in D.C. and all 50 states. The seed money will be provided by the government on the condition that, eventually, the non-profit companies will be financially independent.

To conservatives, the development of a network of non-profit insurance companies looks like a Trojan horse attempting to secretly bring about a public option avoided in the bill. Obviously, here the public option concept has been stretched to include everything beyond the for-profit insurance companies'

---

[*] Letter from CBO director Douglas Elmendorf to House Speaker Nancy Pelosi, March 20, 2010 (quoted in
http://www.cato.org/pubs/wtpapers/BadMedicineWP.pdf).
[†] It is generally believed that American veterans' health care has been covered through the Veteran Administration; however, it is not quite so. Only 8.9 million of the total of 22 million veterans are eligible for VA health benefits. The rest are to be covered through the expanded Medicaid, through private health insurance or stay uninsured. The 2012 Lancet's study estimated that there were over 1 million uninsured veterans; close to a quarter of them – 230,000 – lived in states that have rejected Medicaid expansion.
Universal Health Coverage For US Military Veterans Within Reach, But Many Still Lack Coverage: The Lancet; Nov. 24, 2014:
http://www.sciencedaily.com/releases/2014/11/141124080936.htm.

realm. However, having learned how the best (and "non-socialist") health care systems work (like that in France or Israel), we do know that non-profit, basically government-independent insurance companies could be the foundation of a healthy health care system.

On the other hand, an obvious question arises: How could for-profit and non-profit insurance companies compete in the same insurance space? As you recall, in France they do not compete because the for-profit companies sell only supplemental insurance, while roughly 70% of the health insurance market is served by non-profits. Would not injecting non-profit insurance companies, subsidized by the government, into the otherwise completely for-profit market be, in fact, a Trojan horse that would quickly suffocate for-profit insurance? This issue is quite foggy...

An employer who provides his/her employees with health insurance will have to cover not less than 72.5% of premiums for single individuals and 65% for families. The employer may be eligible for a tax credit. Very small businesses will be directly subsidized through the Exchange. In some cases employees may pay their shares of the coverage through the so-called cafeteria plans[*] from their Health Savings Account, (i.e., before taxes). For those purchasing insurance individually, "affordability credits" may be available. Annual and lifetime coverage limits will be prohibited. (For health insurance subsidies, see[21].)

For retirees over 55 not yet eligible for Medicare, the bill establishes a temporary program that will subsidize 80% of their expenses.

A large amount of money ($8 billion) will be allocated to increase the financing of Community Health Centers, especially in inner cities and rural low-income communities. A new program (financed by grants) will be established to organize and support school-based health clinics.

Among the significant achievements of the ACA are extending parents' coverage to young people age 19 through 26, and covering preventive care. Annual check-ups, mammograms and colonoscopies will be available with no co-payments. Beginning with 2013 most health-care policies covered contraceptives completely.

Health plans may or may not cover abortions: according to the bill, at least one state plan must not include the coverage. Plans using federal funding may cover abortions only if they save a life or are necessary in cases of rape or

---

[*] A cafeteria benefit plan allows an employee to chose from a variety of options to create the most beneficiary combination. The Internal Revenue Code allows qualified cafeteria plans to be tax deductible.

incest. States, however, have the right to prohibit Exchange plans from covering abortions, although interstate plans will be allowed to do so.

Medicaid will be significantly expanded.[8] Previously, only pregnant women and children under age six with an income below 133%FPL were covered, whereas older children: age 8 to18 were covered with family income only up to 100%FPL (some states provided more generous coverage for children above poverty level). Before the Supreme Court decision, the ACA had mandated that all people under age 65 ineligible for Medicare (including children, pregnant women, parents, and adults without dependent children) with modified adjusted gross incomes up to 138%FPL, would be covered by Medicaid. Undocumented immigrants would not be eligible. The guaranteed coverage would "meet the *Essential Health Benefits* available through the Exchanges."

The Supreme Court, however, has found such expansion of Medicaid unconstitutional:[4] the states cannot be forced to accept the burden of sharing the expenses for coverage of millions of new Medicaid enrollees with the federal government. States may or may not agree to the expansion. That, according to a CBO estimate, may significantly increase the number of uninsured.[22]

The states that agree to expand Medicaid enrollment will receive federal financing. In 2013 and 2014 the rate of payment for Medicaid services will be raised to match Medicare payments. The government will completely reimburse states for those expenses. States will also have to enforce the eligibility of children for Medicaid and CHIP and extend the funding through 2015.

As I mentioned, those with income below 400%FPL ($75,200/year for a family of three) who are not eligible for Medicaid will qualify for refundable tax credits to help purchase health insurance through Exchange. Between 2014 and 2020 this subsidy will reach $457 billion.[11]

Medicaid is an entitlement program. It is completely paid for by the federal government and the states. Unlike the "new" Medicaid, which, for a few years will mostly be financed by the government, the financial burden of Medicare will be carried by the elderly.

To begin with, the Medicare A (hospital insurance) the tax rate for incomes above $200,000 and $250,000 for an individual and a family respectively is being raised in 2013 from 1.45% to 2.35%. A new 3.8% tax will also be imposed on capital gains and interest and dividends of high-income earners, applied to the excess of the above incomes.[8] And people with such incomes are not "super rich" anymore; they are solid middle class.

Federal Medicare spending will be cut. The legislation estimates that over 10 years, because of the cuts, the spending will be $417 to $459 billion less.[11] One of the expected is decrease in fee-for-service payments. In 2011 the CBO projected that, "under current law, payment rates for physician services will be reduced by 29.4% in 2012." [23] (As of July 2013, this has not yet happened, although, due to the sequester, the payments have been decreased by 2%.) Among other measures, payments for "bundled services,"[*] where possible, will be substituted for fee-for-service reimbursement. If the cuts are to be achieved by slashing doctors' and hospitals' fees, that may be a disaster for the entire medical system. Among the anticipated cuts are $3 billion for procedures that are believed to be "overused," such as diagnostic screening and imaging. Reimbursement cuts for CT scans or MRI procedures used by seniors began in 2011.[24] Among other cuts is freezing reimbursement rates for health care at home and inpatient rehabilitation. The Medicare B premiums for income earners are being frozen from 2011 through 2019. A positive ACA's initiative: From 2011, 10% bonuses were supposed to be paid to Medicare primary-care physicians and general surgeons working in areas with physician shortages.

A possible $136 billion cut may affect the Medicare Advantage (MA) Program. Medicare Advantage, unlike traditional Medicare, involves private insurers. To many Americans it is a less expensive substitute for Medigap – private supplemental insurance that picks up at least a part of the 20% fees unpaid by Medicare. Some 27% of all those eligible for Medicare (over 13 million) enroll in MA, among them 40% of African Americans and 54% of the Hispanic-speaking elderly. The anticipated increase in premiums may force a significant number of seniors, especially minority seniors, out of MA.[†] On the other hand, a restructuring of MA payments, depending on services and enrollees' age, will introduce some reimbursements as well as payment caps.

The infamous "doughnut hole"[‡] in Medicare D will be gradually patched. Drug manufacturers were required to lower the prices for prescription drugs, providing a 50% discount beginning in 2011; with government subsidies, this

---

[*] Defined as "the reimbursement of health care providers (such as hospitals and physicians) 'on the basis of expected costs for clinically-defined episodes of care.' It has been described as 'a middle ground' between fee-for-service reimbursement (in which providers are paid for each service rendered to a patient) and capitation (in which providers are paid a "lump sum" per patient regardless of how many services the patient receives)." (http://en.wikipedia.org/wiki/Bundled_payment).
[†] "Medicare's chief actuary estimates that more than 7 million seniors could be forced out of their current insurance plan and back into traditional Medicare" (quoted in http://www.cato.org/pubs/wtpapers/BadMedicineWP.pdf).
[‡] When a beneficiary reaches the prescription drug coverage limit, he/she has to pay the entire cost of prescription drugs, until the "catastrophic coverage threshold" has been reached.

---

discount will reach 75% by 2020. In 2010, the one-time doughnut hole rebates of $250 were paid to seniors who had reached the hole. Subsidies for Part D premiums for incomes over $85,000 for individuals and $170,000 for families will be reduced. Tax deductions for retirees who receive drug payment subsidies was to be eliminated in 2013.

Under the 1993 Family and Medical Leave Act, American working women are eligible for 12 weeks of unpaid maternity leave. One could have hoped that the new health care reform would patch that hole. However, my attempts to find in the bill any tangible measures to do with maternity benefits (apart from including maternity riders in new health plans) failed. Only Medicaid and CHIP enrollees will receive such benefits (and no details are provided). It is sad. I will discuss this shameful issue in the next chapter.

Another issue that the new legislation has failed to resolve is long-term health (LTH) care. Until October 15, 2011, the bill did have a provision related to LTH: the Community Living Assistance Services and Support Act (CLASS), originally introduced by Edward Kennedy. CLASS would authorize LTH care for all Americans, who would be automatically enrolled into the program.[25] On October 15, in her letter to senior Democrats and Republicans in Congress, Secretary of Health and Human Services Kathleen Sebelius stated that the CLASS program could not be financially sustainable.[26] I will discuss this issue in the next chapter.

As a federal reform, ACA mandates the states to comply with its requirements. An important requirement is that each state has to decide on a benchmark insurance plan that would provide essential health benefits. As of December 2012, all states did that.[27]

Let me turn now to the second key objective of Obamacare:

Stop insurance discriminating practices.

According to the bill, all kinds of discriminating practices based on pre-existing physical or mental conditions, gender or health status, genetic information, and so forth are prohibited.

Although the premiums should be the same in the same class of insured, they can vary depending on some conditions. For example, a smoker will have to pay up to 50% more than a non-smoker. Premiums may also vary with age; however, they cannot be more that three times higher for older people than for the young.

The prohibition against health discrimination does not come into force immediately. Most probably insurance companies could not afford to lose such a big chunk of profit right away. The government agreed. Therefore, as a temporary measure (till 2014), the so-called "national high-risk pool" will be established. In order to be enrolled, a person with pre-existing medical conditions has to be refused coverage for at least six months (!). The premiums for those in the pool may be high, so some will be eligible for government subsidies. The discrimination of children was prohibited right away.

The third objective:

Bring down the cost of health insurance by slashing bureaucracy.

The new ACA bureaucracy is enormous. Here is a partial list of programs, advisory boards, innovation centers, etc.[2,8]

- *Health Choices Administration.* This administration's tzar, the Commissioner, would oversee a national health insurance Exchange in which Americans theoretically could purchase affordable coverage. That would include the establishment of qualified health benefits plan standards, along with the enforcement of such standards in coordination with State insurance regulators and the Secretaries of Labor and the Treasury.

- *Independent Payment Advisory Board* comprised of 15 members to submit legislative proposals containing recommendations to reduce per capita rate of growth in Medicare spending if spending exceeds a target growth rate. The most heavily criticized IPAB's legislation is reimbursing physicians for discussing with patients and their relatives optimal strategies of end-of-life treatments. (That is why IPAB is often referred to by conservatives as the Death Panel.) I will discuss this issue in the next chapter.

- *Innovation Center Within the Centers for Medicare and Medicaid Services* to test, evaluate, and expand in Medicare, Medicaid, and CHIP different payment structures and methodologies to reduce program expenditures while maintaining or improving quality of care.

- *Patient-Centered Outcomes Research Institute* to identify research priorities and conduct research that compares the clinical effectiveness of medical treatments. This Institute will be overseen by an appointed multi-stakeholder board of governors and will be assisted by expert advisory panels (two more bureaucratic bodies!).

- *National Health Care Workforce Commission* to develop a national work force strategy.

- Task forces on *Preventive Services and Community Preventive Services* to develop, update, and disseminate evidenced-based recommendations on the use of clinical and community prevention services.

• *National Prevention, Health Promotion, and Public Health Council* for prevention, wellness, and public health activities including prevention research and health screenings, the Education and Outreach Campaign for preventive benefits, and immunization programs. It will be financed by a $13 billion Trust Fund, and will establish a grant program to support the delivery of evidence-based and community-based prevention and wellness services aimed at strengthening prevention activities, reducing chronic disease rates, and addressing health disparities, especially in rural and frontier areas.

• *Community-based Collaborative Care Network Program* to support consortiums of health care providers to coordinate and integrate health care services for low-income uninsured and underinsured populations.

• *White House Council on Women and Girls* to develop "policies that establish a balance between work and family."

Each of those organizations and boards may do useful work in improving health care. However, it is unlikely that their functioning would decrease the ACA's financial burden on American economy. However, they will definitely strengthen multi-faceted government control of health care.

Here I would like to make a note. Before the final House Bill H.R. 3962 was signed into law, there existed Senate Bill H.R. 3590, which is no longer a valid document. Its Section 2510 contained the provision of establishing a *Commissioned Ready Reserve Corps*, which has been interpreted by Obamacare critics as a paramilitary force directly under the President's command. It is probably because of this controversy that this clause has not been included in the final Bill H.R. 3590. What I would like to clarify is that the *Commissioned Ready Reserve Corps* does exist as a military entity irrespective of the ACA. These are rapidly deployed units consisting of 6,500 full time officers, doctors, and other medical personnel to be used in extreme situations under direct orders from the President.

> Over the last few years, Commissioned Corps officers have provided leadership and humanitarian health services during several natural disasters, such as the Indian Ocean Tsunami of 2004, Hurricanes Katrina and Rita in 2005, and Hurricanes Ike and Gustav in 2008. They have also provided support during the 2001 anthrax attacks and after the attack on the World Trade Center.[28]

Obviously such a force is necessary. The objective of including that provision into health care bill had probably been to strengthen the force: to extend it and to make it more "military." The participants would be expected to participate in routine military training, and, although the Corps is voluntarily, the officers might be called to active duty in any emergency.

The fourth reform objective that I mentioned above deals with

Eliminating Fraud and Abuse.

Here, in a nutshell, are the measures to be taken in order to achieve that goal:[29]

> • Increase funding by $100 million annually for the Health Care Fraud and Abuse Control Fund to fight Medicare and Medicaid fraud;
>
> • Improve provider and payment screening to prevent fraud and abuse before it occurs;
>
> • Create enhanced oversight for Medicare and Medicaid programs at risk of fraud and abuse;
>
> • Create new penalties for providers and suppliers that defraud federal health care programs;
>
> • Partner with the private sector to reduce waste and abuse by requiring that all Medicare and Medicaid providers establish compliance programs to reduce waste, fraud, and abuse.

In the next section I will discuss fraud and abuse in Medicaid, Medicare and the health care system as a whole. It would be great if all the above measures were implemented. However, overcharging those who can pay the bills (making up for those who cannot) is a popular form of abuse inherent in the system where health care is a commodity, and, as such may have different prices depending, partly, on the integrity of health-care providers.

Let me summarize the most important ACA factors.

Coverage (the RAND[*] analysis[10] and Census Bureau data [14]):

> • The main goal of the reform, *No Uninsured Left Behind*, will not be achieved.
>
> Among some 20+ million left uninsured are 5 million youngsters who will not be covered through their parents and 12 million who are

---

[*] RAND (**R**esearch **AN**d **D**evelopment) Corporation is a nonprofit, non-partisan international think tank financed mostly by the U.S. government and other private sources. The analysis I am quoting from has been done using the RAND COMPARE computer model.

unlucky enough to live in states that refused to expand Medicaid to 138%FPL. Some people will probably decide to pay a penalty rather than purchase insurance.

Among those who will be covered are: 3 million young people age 19-26, through their parents' insurance; approximately half of people with income between 100%FPL and 138%FPL who will get access to Medicaid in states that would agree to expand Medicaid coverage – some 12 million; and about 9 million people who will be covered in spite of pre-existing conditions. This adds up to 24 million. Others with incomes between 138%FPL and 400%FPL will be able to purchase insurance, thanks to government subsidies. The RAND Corporation estimates that 56% of those previously uninsured will be covered, equaling some 27 million (based on Census Bureau 's 48.6 million uninsured).

• Those without insurance in 2019 will be younger, healthier, and wealthier than we would expect in the absence of the policy changes.

• Compared with the projected status-quo trend, by 2019, about 12 million more people will be enrolled in employer-sponsored insurance, 12 million more (16-24 million by CBO estimates) in Medicaid, and 8 million more in non-group insurance through an Exchange.

Spending (RAND[10])

• The estimated $753 billion cumulative increase in personal health spending between 2010 and 2019 represents an increase of 3.3% over the status-quo projection.

• Between 2010 and 2019, cumulative federal spending on subsidies for those who obtain insurance through the Exchange will be $445 billion. Approximately 53% of the 25 million people purchasing insurance through the Exchange in 2019 will receive a federal subsidy.

• Medicaid spending is projected to increase by $559 billion between 2010 and 2019, a 21% increase over the projected trend in the status-quo.

• Penalty payments for those not complying with the mandates will total $75 billion from individuals and $108 billion from employers between 2013 and 2019.

• In 2019, average insurance premiums in the large group (employer) market will be at least 2% lower than projected in the status-quo.

• There will be some increase in insurance premiums for the most common non-group policies. The increase is higher in the first few years after the reform (8%) and becomes negligible by 2019, with an average increase over the whole period of about 4%. When the market stabilizes (2016–2019), the premiums will be about 2% higher than would have been observed in the non-group market without the policy change. The presence of subsidies will further soften the effect of this increase on the population.

Those families earning $18,000 (about 100%FPL) per year will not see any financial gains because of Medicaid assistance. The net income of those earning $18,000 – $55,000 (about 300%FPL) per year will increase roughly by $2,000. For those in the top 1% of income (more than $348,000 per year) the new taxes and reduced benefits will cost on average some $52,000 more.[11]

Funding (Obamacare Facts [7])

The main sources of revenue will be taxes, fees, and penalties. Officially, the new taxes will supply $409.2 billion over 10 years. Here is a brief summary of the revenue sources:

• Increase Medicare tax by 0.9% for those earning more than $200,000 and $250,000, for individual and joint filers respectively: $210.2 billion

• Annual fee on health insurance providers: $60 billion

• 40% excise tax on health care policies in excess of $10,200/$27,500: $32 billion

• Annual fee on manufacturers and importers of branded drugs: $27 billion

• 2.3% excise tax on manufacturers and importers of certain medical devices: $20 billion

• Requirement of information reporting on payments to insurance companies:[*] $17.1 billion

• Limit health flexible spending arrangements in cafeteria plans: $13 billion

• All other revenue sources: $14.9 billion

---

[*] Beginning in 2012, a business has to send a Form 1099-Miss to insurance company it deals with, thus preventing the latter from not paying taxes on the payments.

From 2013 one will be allowed to deduct medical expenses above 10% of adjusted gross income rather than 7.5% before the reform (for those 65 and older the new threshold will be enforced in 2016). This will bring $15.2 billion more.

Actually, the ACA's Title IX, the Revenue Provisions, provides financing for only half the cost of the ACA. *As for the rest, about $450 billion, it will be provided by "savings from lowering Medicare's rate of growth" between 2010 and 2019 (Title III)*; e.g. cutting Medicare financing, which means that the elderly will have to carry a significant Obamacare load.

Let me now summarize the current and nearest future ACA progress:[30,31] *

In 2012:
• Insurance companies must cover dependents up to age 26 and children under 19 regardless of pre-existing conditions.
• No lifetime limit on essential benefits.
• No co-payments for preventive care: physical examination, mammogram, contraceptives.

In 2013:
• Begin establishment of American Health Benefit Exchanges
• New limits on tax-free contributions to Health Savings Account: $3,250 for individuals and $6,450 for families.
• 0.9% increase of payroll Medicare tax for high wage earners.
• 2.3% excise tax on medical devices begins.
• The threshold at which medical expenses as a percentage of income become deductible increases to 10% from 7.5%.

Starting in 2014:
• Complete establishing American Health Benefit Exchanges
• Employees with 50 or more full-time workers if they don't offer insurance could pay $2,000 penalty per employee, excluding the first 30 employees.
• Waiting periods over 90 days for policies provided by employers will be prohibited.
• Employers with a full-time staff of more than 200 must automatically enroll new workers in a health care plan.
• An individual mandate tax imposed on those refusing to purchase a government-approved coverage (formerly "penalty") begins.
• Pre-existing conditions discrimination is completely prohibited.
• Essential health benefits plans become operational.
• The premium tax credits and cost-sharing assistance begins.

---

* Just for fun: one can take an "ACA Quiz:"
http://healthreform.kff.org/quizzes/health-reform-quiz/question-1.aspx.

For projected ACA development beyond 2014 see.[31]

In March 2014, as I am updating this chapter, there are already some outcomes of the first Obamacare steps: [32,33]

•Thirty-one per cent of physicians experience an increase in the number of their patients, though sometimes with increasing waiting time. They see the return of patients who have previously dropped out because of insurance costs. Forty per cent of doctors do not experience an increase in patients.

•Seventy-one percent of physicians accept Medicaid and Medicare patients; 3% accept Medicare but not Medicaid patients; 11% do not accept and do not intend to accept such patients. In Medicare Advantage plans, doctors' reimbursement is almost one half that of Medicare; some doctors are expected to stop participating with these plans. Slash of payments to Medicare physicians is expected. If it happens, more physicians will leave Medicare.

•Many Americans, having signed up for Obamacare, have access to limited groups of doctors and hospitals. Doctors who previously treated a patient become unavailable. Switching to a higher "tier," say from a Bronze to a Silver plan, may help with increase of deductibles and co-pays.

There are endless discussions in Congress and in the media of whether the new health care reform will decrease or increase the deficit. I do not want to be involved in this strongly partisan argument. The future will determine the outcome.

As I mentioned in the first chapter, a number of states have developed or have been developing their own health care systems prior to the ACA. As of 2009, three states, Maine, Massachusetts and Vermont, implemented their own reforms that achieved almost universal coverage of their residents. At that time 14 more states were considering comprehensive reforms. Because some ACA rules are different from those implemented in the states' systems, there are conflicts.

The Massachusetts law was passed under the governorship of Mitt Romney in 2006 and quickly became popular.* It was completely operational by 2009 and was quite successful: by 2008, the number of uninsured fell from 14% of

---

* In the 2010 midterm elections something unprecedented for Massachusetts happened: a Republican, Scott Brown, was elected to the Senate to take the Edward Kennedy's seat. Was it because, all of a sudden, Massachusetts became conservative? Very unlikely. Most probably, the people of Massachusetts decided that they do not need a new and Washington-controlled health plan while they do have their own, and a *good* one. In 2012 the momentum was lost and Scott Brown was not re-elected. Massachusetts is still a loyal Democratic state.

residents to 6%.

Massachusetts is my home, and I would like to say just a few words about its health care system. Although Romneycare, as it is often called, most probably was a blueprint for Obamacare, the two are different. To begin with, it is a state program, whereas the ACA, although it delegates some functions to states, is directed by the federal administration. Some ACA provisions are binding even if states disagree with them. Here are some Romneycare features compared with Obamacare (for more details see:[34])

• As with Obamacare, Massachusetts residents had to obey the individual mandate that required adult residents to have health insurance. The legislated minimum preventive coverage included preventive and primary care, emergency services, hospitalization benefits, ambulatory patient services, mental health services and prescription drug coverage. Failure to purchase insurance resulted in a tax penalty, which was more severe than in Obamacare and discouraged people from remaining outside the system.

•The employer mandate required employers with more than 50 employees to provide insurance for them. The penalty for failing to do so was $295 per employee/per year. The Obamacare penalty structure is more complex (see above).

• As with Obamacare, residents were purchasing health insurance online through Commonwealth Health Insurance Connector – called Exchanges in Obamacare.

• Medicaid[*] eligibility was extended more than in Obamacare: to children below 300% of FPL, and to adults below 150% (Obamacare extends Medicaid to 138%FPL). For those ineligible for Medicaid within 150%-300% FPL, subsidies were available.

• Under Romneycare young adults up to age 26 could purchase a reduced benefits policy through Connector if they do not have insurance through employers. Obamacare authorizes young adults up to age 26 and children under 19 to be covered by their parents' policies irrespective of pre-existing conditions or their possible coverage through employers.

Because some Obamacare provisions seriously disagree with the Massachusetts law, "it is not clear how conflicts will be resolved."[35]

For detailed information on the other states' "would-be" health care reforms, see.[36]

---

[*] Medicaid combined with CHIP is called "Masshealth" in Massachusetts.

* * *

H.R. 3962 begins with a statement claiming that the new health care reform is not a revolution: It is "building on what works in today's health care system, while repairing the aspects that are broken."

However, it is the most significant change in the American health care system since Medicaid and Medicare were created. As someone living in Massachusetts, I feel very keenly that the long-awaited "health care for all" would have been more popular and more successful were it based on a conglomerate of states' own plans, which had already been gradually emerging. That opportunity has been lost. The ACA will remain in place, possibly for a long time. Whether the reform survives future political battles or not, it will have significant impact on America's health care system.

4. WHERE ARE WE?

America's Health Care Today

> Sherlock Holmes and Dr. Watson fly in a
> balloon and have lost their way. They
> descend and see a man with a laptop.
> –Where are we? asks Dr. Watson.
> – In a balloon.
> –Are you a programmer? asks Sherlock
> Holmes.
> –No, sir. I am a peasant.
>
> *An Internet joke*

Where are we now?

Remember the famous quote from William Shakespeare's *Hamlet*: "Something is rotten in the state of Denmark"? We do know that *something is rotten* in our health care. In this chapter I will not be discussing the millions of uninsured: Obama reform has dealt with that, albeit not quite successfully. I will attempt to reflect on other "somethings," which Obamacare has not touched, not pretending that my understanding of the problems is absolutely right – just as something to think about.

A British blogger believes that any reconstruction of the U.S. health system needs to begin with the simple question: "Where the f- is all that money going?"[1] Unless you can answer that and stop the rot, you'll have the same problems regardless of having universal health care or not.

This is a popular view. However, as we shall see, it is not quite right. And it is "rotting money" that I would like to discuss.

But first, a short reflection on our overspending.

As I mentioned previously, the U.S. has the highest percentage of GDP spent on health care among all the OECD countries: 17.7 %. You can see from the table in the last chapter that the total health expenditure per capita in the U.S. – $8,508 – is almost twice as high as that of the six other countries. The money

Where Are We?

Americans pay out of pocket* – $987.4 – is also the highest: Canada, with $669.6, is the closest; in the other countries patients pay significantly less (because their health insurance pays more).

Total Health Expenditure Per Capita and GDP Per Capita: US and Selected Countries, 2008[†]

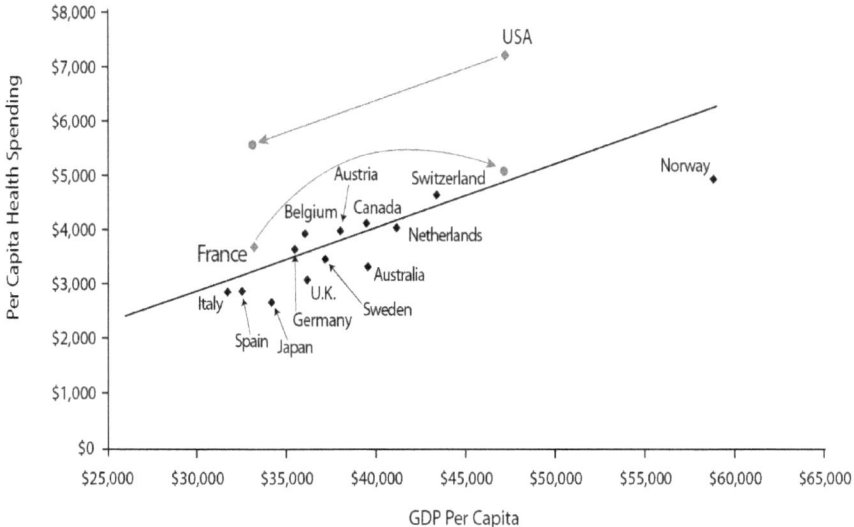

The OECD graph above[2] shows the relationship between GDP per capita and health care expenditure by various countries. The solid line is the closest fit of the scattered diamonds representing different OECD countries. The U.S. diamond does not belong on that line. We see that all the non-U.S. diamonds cluster more or less smoothly along the line. Let us call it "living according to one's means."

Our health care spending is much higher: it is almost 60% more than the curve would "predict"; it is as if Americans decided to purchase only Porsches and Mercedeses, which we cannot afford.

On the other hand, it is obvious that the richer the nation the more people

---

* Paid directly by a patient when insurance does not cover the full cost of service. These costs include all co-payments, costs for any medications, and other health care expenditures.
† Organization for Economic Co-operation and Development (2010), "OECD Health Data," *OECD Health Statistics* (database) (Accessed on February 14, 2011). Data from Australia and Japan are from 2007. Figures for Belgium, Canada, Netherlands, Norway and Switzerland are OECD estimates. This graph is only for illustration; more recent data would not change it significantly.

spend. Therefore it is not unexpected that the U.S., with the highest GDP, spends more than the other nations on health care. We also spend more on cars and entertainment. Nobody forces Americans to buy expensive SUVs or expensive subscriptions for hundreds of TV channels. We do it because we believe that we *can afford* it. Taking this into account, how much more do we *actually* spend on health care than the other countries?

If we take the ratio of our GDP per capita and that of, say, France (from the horizontal axis of the plot below, or slightly different entries in the table in next chapter), we will see that even if we did not drive Mercedeses and lived according to our means (e.g., our health care expenses were somewhere close to the solid line) we would have to pay our doctors close to 1.4 times more than the French pay their doctors. If one compares the 2011 disposable (after taxes) incomes in the U.S. ($40,916) and France ($29,436)[3] one can see that Americans have 1.39 times more money to spend (including on health care) than the French have. It is almost the same factor of 1.4. If we compare our health care expenses with those of France, the factor will be about 2. If we now take France as a role model and see how much we would pay for health care, being 1.4 times less rich, our spending per capita would be $5,500, and we would find ourselves on the diagram (see a fat circle that I have added above France's diamond) only about 50% higher, rather than 100% higher. Yet, we are still rather high above that curve. On the other hand, if France were as affluent as we are (i.e., if its GDP per capita were about 1.4 times higher), its spending per capita would be about $5,400, and its fat circle would sit below the U.S.'s diamond but very close to the curve. So, they would be more or less OK.

To make the idea more generally applicable, in the last chapter I introduced an *Affluence Factor*: the ratio of the U.S. GDP per capita to those of other countries. It varies from 1.25 (Canada) to 1.73 (Israel) with France (1.43) in between (see the table there; I will be referring to it as "the table"). If we want to compare how much the U.S. spends on health care with other countries, we have to compare "apples to apples," that is, we have to compare spending not just in U.S. dollars but in "true" dollars, multiplying the statistical health care expenses of each country by its *Affluence Factor*, and then comparing them with what Americans spend. Then we could compare our expenses with those of other countries, assuming them to be as affluent as we are. As one can see from the table, things are not so gloomy, but gloomy enough.

A May 2012 analysis of health care spending in the U.S. and OECD countries commissioned by the Commonwealth Fund finds that in the U.S. it is more likely that higher spending "is largely due to higher prices and perhaps more readily accessible technology and greater obesity."[4]

Now let us try to see where we are overspending.

"Money Rotting"

We saw that the main difference between our health care system and those in the other six countries is that ours is run mostly by for-profit insurance companies, which, as people firmly believe, make huge profits and award their CEOs fat bonuses.

So the first suspicion is that the health insurers are the villains responsible for our health care ills. What is "a huge profit"? As an economist would say, a profit is quantitatively expressed by a "profit margin." It is a percentage of the money made relative to the total money spent on salaries, including CEO bonuses, advertising, and the various expenses that any company has. I was astonished to learn that health insurance companies' typical profit margin, as we will see from the list below, is quite low. The median is only 3.7%. In contrast, pharmaceutical companies' profits are much higher: 16.4% (2010)[5]. Here is a list comparing the 2009 profit margins of health insurance companies:[6]

Net Profit Margin of Health care Insurers:

> Aetna: 3.7%
> Wellpoint: 7.3%
> Cigna: 7.1%
> United Health: 3.7%
> Humana: 3.4%
> Healthnet: -0.3%
> Healthspring: 5.0%
> Coventry Health Care: 2.3%
> Molina Health Care: 0.8%
> United American Corp: 2.7%
> Unum Group: 8.4%
> And I add here Blue Cross Blue Shield's 0.0%

For comparison:
Net Profit Margin of Internet/Tech Companies (median: 13.1%):
> Google: 27.6%
> Yahoo: 9.2%
> Microsoft: 24.9%
> Baidu: 4.8%
> Apple: 19.2%
> AOL: 7.6%

Nokia: 3.0%
Adobe: 13.1%
Sohu: 28.6%

Health insurers' rank by profit margin among commercial companies is No. 88, and they make on average between $100 and $200 per policy.[7] Multiply that by a hundred million policies, and you will see that even with relatively low profit margin they do afford both paying high bonuses and building the highest skyscrapers in town. Thus, the claim that they make a great deal of money does make sense.

However, are the insurance companies the villains that suck up our health care money? Take, for example, Marriott hotels. Their profit margin is quite volatile, and within the last five years the maximum was just 6.63%, and yet they do make a great deal of money.[8] Should we accuse successful businesses and rich people of being bloodsuckers? That would smack of socialist class warfare rhetoric. For-profit health insurance companies are just successful businesses with a low profit margin. Are they completely exonerated?

The answer is not that simple. Insurance companies decide which medical treatments are allowed, which are not, and how much they want to pay for services. In this respect thea are the villain that makes our health care inefficient.

Even if some insurance companies are more efficient than others in juggling our money, their competition has virtually nothing to do with our health, whether they have large or small profits or none at all. We see that the amount of money they make and the bonuses they pay are irrelevant if we want to understand the commercial insurance companies' role in our health care.

Administrative expenses are another factor to examine. Economist Henry Aaron, in his 2003 *New England Journal of Medicine* article, wrote:[9]

> Like many other observers, I look at the U.S. health care system and see an administrative monstrosity, a truly bizarre mélange of thousands of payers with payment systems that differ for no socially beneficial reason, as well as a staggeringly complex public system with mind-boggling administered prices and other rules expressing distinctions that can only be regarded as weird.

He compared administrative expenses in the U.S. and Canada. Nothing has changed in 10 years. The 2013 Medscape Physician Compensation Report[10] found that:

> Doctors are drowning in paperwork, whether it's actual paper or

computer-based reporting. A lucky 20% of respondents have less than 5 hours of paperwork per week, but 51% of physicians spend from 5 to 14 hours per week on paperwork. Another 17% spend more than 20 hours per week on such tasks. And annually, in order to confirm credentials, a physician has to submit nearly 18 different forms.

Administrative costs are enormous: about $360 billion (as of 2012), which is 13.5% of our total health care expenses ($2,640 billion).[11] Of that amount, 85% is due to a complex system of private insurance and its enormous bureaucracies. For every two doctors in the U.S., there is now one health-insurance employee.

Government programs Medicare, Medicaid, Program CHIP, and the Veterans Administration are accused of spending a lot on shuffling papers. However, this is probably not true. According to the Kaiser Family Foundation's data, Medicare's administrative expenses are about 5%.[12] Medicaid's administrative expenses are higher: some 6.5%,[13] but still much lower than those of private insurers.

One of the objectives of the Obamacare reform was to slash administrative expenses. In the chapter on that reform I composed a list of numerous committees and boards that are intended to supervise the new health care system and make it less expensive. As I mentioned, I do not believe that an expanding bureaucracy can ever cut costs. However, even if we forget about the enormous bureaucracy of hundreds of insurance companies (and nothing can be done about that for as long as they run the show) computerization of paperwork could make a tremendous difference.

Europe is far ahead of us but could have been behind if Richard Nixon's health care reform had been implemented 40 years ago. That is what he proposed:[14]

> Every American who participates in the program would receive a Health-card when the plan goes into effect in his state. This card, similar to a credit card, would be honored by hospitals, nursing homes, emergency rooms, doctors, and clinics across the country. This card could also be used to identify information on blood type and sensitivity to particular drugs—information, which might be important in an emergency. Bills for the services paid for with the Health-card would be sent to the insurance carrier who would reimburse the provider of the care for covered services, then bill the patient for his share, if any.

Nixon's suggestion was ahead of its time: personal computers had not yet conquered the world. Over quarter of a century later, a decade ago, European countries began using a medical card that identified patients and made all monetary transactions digital. French Card Vitale has been used since 1998; as a result, French clinics and hospitals have 67% fewer people in administrative offices than comparable institutions in the U.S.[15] Taiwan, which has been using a Smart Card since 1995, spends only 2% of its total health care costs on administrative expenses.

For a decade, a joint business and government group, the *Smart Card Alliance*, has been advancing the development of the Smart Card in America, and not only in medicine.[16] The main reasons America still does not have the Smart Card is our fragmented health care system, with an enormous number of independent medical establishments, and the impossibility of imposing radical changes in a centralized way. Even though centralization in general is bad, the health card has to be uniform, as uniform as our driving license. President Obama's Stimulus Package assigned $19 billion towards "utilization of an electronic health record for each person in the United States by 2014."[17] However, according to Randy Vanderhoof, director of the *Smart Card Alliance*, Smart Cards "have a long way to go. They can't happen overnight in a system that's both fundamentally broken and going through major upheaval." He estimates that we will have to wait about a decade before the Smart Card conquers our health care system.*

Medical cards used in other countries do not contain any medical information, the addition of which would significantly facilitate physicians' work. A card that contains all the information on the patient's health: when and which physicians are seen, diagnoses, test results, EKG, X-ray, MRI, CT scan and other procedures' results may appear soon. Security of access to that information is probably the main issue (suppose the card has been lost or stolen?). Meanwhile, computerization of patients' medical files is spreading in the U.S. Lack of centralization is the major obstacle. In the Greater Boston area, all the doctors and hospitals that belong to *Partners* – a consortium of major Boston hospitals – have access to their patients' files on line; patients also have access to their files. Those who do not belong do not have access to that important information.

The next suspicion about "money rotting" is that compared to other countries, we allegedly grossly overpay for drugs. Unlike other countries, we pay

---

* Meanwhile, "According to the General Services Administration (the government's accounting arm), as many as 90% of all decisions made by Medicare on whether services are medically necessary are made by workers with only high school educations and no medical training or background. At the rate of 400 claims per worker per day – 1 claim every 72 seconds – it's no wonder they make so many mistakes"
(http://www.medscape.com/viewarticle/754422?src=mp). Would not a Smart Card do the job better?

pharmaceutical companies what they ask. Medicare, for instance, is even prohibited by law to negotiate drug prices. However, again, having multiplied the pharmaceutical expenses of other countries by their *Affluence Factors*, we see that the difference between what they and we spend is not huge (see the table). In the case of France, it is just 8%, rather than 64% as "uncorrected" statistics claim.

On the other hand, an avalanche of new and efficient drugs pushes their prices up because the prices also include the cost of pharmaceutical research. The cost of brand name drugs are on average 75% higher that that of generic drugs, which typically remain the same from 7 to 12 years until the patent for the drug expires. Over 50% of prescribed drugs are generic. Just recently, Lipitor (atorvastatin), an efficient cholesterol-controlling drug, has become generic.

An important factor in health care cost is the development of state-of-the-art medical technologies and procedures. The U.S. is the pioneer in this field.[*] The National Institute of Health (NIH) plays a significant role in transferring new technologies to private businesses.

The next suspicion of why American health care is so expensive is high physicians' fees. Let me quote from[18]:

> Actually, let's split that question in two. The first is whether U.S. doctors are overpaid. The second is whether paying them less would save all that much. The answers, respectively: yes and no.

Upon closer examination, however, the first answer also happens to be NO. First of all, as I illustrated on the plot above discussing our health care expenses, American doctors are supposed to be paid more than in other countries simply because our GDP per capita is higher. We pay doctors more than the French, but not much more than the 1.4 *Affluence Factor*. In 2009, for general practitioners it was roughly 1.75 (on average we paid $161,000/year against $92,000 in France). For specialists, the difference is even smaller: 1.54 ($230,000 against $149,000).[†19] It is difficult to estimate physicians' "average" incomes. In 2012, family doctors earned annually more than in 2009: $175,000; about one third of physician specialties earned $300,000 (the three top were orthopedists – $405,000, cardiologists – $357,000, and radiologists – $349,000); the lowest salaried were pediatrics and HIV/ID doctors, respectively $173,000 and $170,000.[10]

We already see that the overpayment of doctors in America comes into

---

[*] Probably sharing the first place with Israel.
[†] Unfortunately, I could not find on the Internet data on "physician compensation worldwide" for later years.

question. Before going into detailed analysis, I would like to note that, even disregarding the "driving Mercedeses" syndrome, doctors' fees must be drawn up by market mechanisms. As one can see from the table, we have a shortage of doctors: 2.5 per 1000 population, which is below France (3.3), Germany (3.8), and Israel (3.3). The supply of doctors does not satisfy the demand for their services; hence their higher fees. We typically do not have to wait for a specialist appointment for months but a few weeks is not unusual, and the fees are high because there is virtually no competition for patients among doctors.

The shortage of primary care physicians (PCP) is an even more serious issue because they are on the forefront of health care. Primary care physicians are underpaid even comparing with the lowest paid specialists. Only highly idealistic medical students choose to become internists. In order to see more patients PCPs have had to shrink their appointment times from 20 minutes to 10, and sometimes even less. As a result, they do not have enough time to evaluate patients' complains thoroughly. A study showed that "Patients receive only 55% of recommended chronic and preventive services."[*20] Therefore they "abuse" referring their patients to specialists, and this costs our health care billions. More and more often, a nurse practitioner substitutes for a doctor, even in emergency situations requiring high competence. When a patient has coughing symptoms and the nurse practitioner prescribes an antibiotic without sending the patient for an X-ray (and I do know of cases like that) it is wrong and may be dangerous. According to the Association of American Medical Colleges,[21] by 2020, the shortage of doctors will reach 91,000: 46,000 surgeons and specialists, and 45,000 primary care physicians. Medical schools have a goal to increase students' enrollment by 30 percent by 2016. However, a shortage of federally funded residency positions for new doctors is looming. The National Resident Matching Program (NRMP) helps to find residency placement for graduates. However, "According to the NRMP, last year [2011] 971 graduates of U.S. medical schools were shut out, accounting for 5.9% of

---

[*] This study estimated that in order for a group of doctors who share their clinic ("a health–care team") to be economically viable, each PCP has to have a so-called "physician panel"– the total number of patients under his/her care – of about 2000 patients. The panel size depends on how much time is needed per patient for preventive, chronic, and acute services. In one example, if a doctor spends 10 min/patient/year for preventive care; 32 min. for chronic care, and 22 min. for acute care (the total of 64 min/patient/year), the panel size consists of 1,947 patients. Other source claims that an "ideal panel" should consist of 1806 patients, provided that a patient sees PCP 3.19 times/year, and the doctor sees 24 patients/day, working for 240 days/year. *(Panel Size: How many Patients can one doctor manage?:*http://www.aafp.org/fpm/2007/0400/p44.html#fpm20070400p44-bt2). We see that the time and ability to render a high quality care by a PCP is squeezed to an almost impossible degree.

U.S. grads. Graduates of international medical schools fared even worse - less than 50% of them obtained a residency. That means more than 7,000 doctors were left with a diploma that said 'M.D.' but no guarantee they would be able to use it."[22].

At the same time, the residents who have been lucky to find a hospital work like slaves: their workweeks sometimes reach 80 hours.* They are overstressed and burned out. No wonder, "Suicide accounts for 26 percent of deaths among physicians aged 25 to 39, as compared to 11 percent of deaths in the same age group in the general population."[23] The suicide rate of physicians of all ages is estimated to be between 1.4-2.3 times the rate in the general population: "It has been reliably estimated that on average the United States loses as many as 400 physicians to suicide each year (the equivalent of at least one entire medical school)."[24]

Since 1997, federal funding for residency training has not been increasing, and the situation will hardly be improved because of budget cuts.

Compared to the average (or "mean") income of Americans, our doctors make about 5.5 times more. We also pay physicians more than they pay in other countries. For example, the corresponding ratios in Canada, France, Germany, and Great Britain are 3.2, 1.9, 3.4, and 1.4.[18] But are our doctors "overpaid"?

An American doctor needs to be compensated with a higher income for several reasons. On average, having graduated from medical school, American doctors carry debts of no less than $150,000–$200,000.† Add to that the debt accumulated during four years of undergraduate studies even not at an Ivy League university. As we saw in France, Germany, and Britain, medical schools are free (or almost free) and an undergraduate diploma is not necessary in order to be accepted to a medical school because the high schools there provide sufficient preparation for medical studies.‡ Like almost every problem

---

* In 2003, "The Accreditation Council for Graduate Medical Education (ACGME) has limited the number of workhours to 80 hours weekly, overnight call frequency to no more than one in three, 30-hour maximum straight shifts, and at least 10 hours off between shifts." "The U.S. Occupational Safety and Health Administration (OSHA) rejected a petition seeking to restrict medical resident work hours." (*Medical resident work hours:* http://en.wikipedia.org/wiki/medical_resident_work_hours#cite_note-6). Compare it with the European Union's regulation that a medical resident did not have to work more than 48 hours a week.
† My friends' son, now in his second year of medical school, who refuses any help from his parents, borrows close to $80,000 every year (tuition plus living expenses). His debt upon graduation may be over $300,000.
‡ Let me again quote from Dr. John Silber's book *Straight Shooting. What Is Wrong With America And How To Fix It*: "At the present moment, I believe very few

in America, our dysfunctional educational system is to blame. We do know that our high school education does not provide even basic knowledge about the world – forget about physics or chemistry. Our students fail miserably in international competitions.

A young American medical doctor faces at least three years of residency with a meager salary of $50,000 and an enormous workload: 80 hours/week is the legal limit. No wonder that having eventually received an M.D. diploma, one wants to earn at least enough to begin paying off the debt.

Even if one is not motivated to become a physician mainly to get rich (unfortunately, there are many doctors of this ilk who had hesitated whether to go to a medical or a law school) – one considers long years of medical studies as a *capital*, which will bring dividends. And not only that. Physicians work hard and have high responsibility for the wellbeing of their patients. They need to be up to date on new developments in their fields and basic science. They have to be able to validate their status by completing periodic continuing education courses. There is nothing immoral in physicians' desire to earn a high income. It is a normal aspiration, especially in a society that respects and rewards people of high financial standing.

Doctors' gross earnings differ significantly from what they bring home. They have to pay for their offices and for malpractice insurance – a total of close to half of their income after taxes.

Typically, a doctor belongs to an association of a few physicians who jointly rent offices, hire the necessary medical personnel and administrative assistants, and pay all the business expenses. It gets increasingly difficult for such small businesses to survive, considering that doctors still need to bring home enough money to pay bills and support their families.

Both private doctors and hospitals have skewed economics. Increasingly, more patients pay by skinny Medicaid checks. The ACA reform lifts the ceiling of eligibility for Medicaid, which, in spite of the restrictions imposed by the Supreme Court, still add some 16 million new patients to Medicaid. [25] The checks of Medicare patients are a bit fatter; however, Medicare pays, on average, less than half of doctors' and hospitals' bills (even less for surgeries and diagnostic tests like MRI and CT scans). How can doctors (and hospitals) escape bankruptcy? Some doctors just leave the game. Increasingly more refuse to accept Medicaid patients. Most doctors, however, cannot afford to reject the elderly: virtually all doctors accept Medicare payments (although psychiatrists are leaving Medicare in droves).

[American] college graduates could pass the A-Level examinations required in England of students who wish merely to enter the university."

Where Are We?

At least three mechanisms exist to enhance doctors' incomes: increase the number of patients they see (a typical doctor's appointment time is 15-20 minutes and is even shorter for PCP's visits, or when a specialty doctor at a follow-up appointment first sends a physician's assistant to see the patient, and then visits the patient often for just a few minutes); have patients undergo more tests (those that the physician's office can provide); and, overcharge the non-Medicaid and non-Medicare patients who have insurance. That is why Americans who are not poor and not old pay more to doctors. Hospitals (including emergency rooms) cannot refuse a patient, and cannot treat people above their bed capacity. But they can and do overcharge those who have health insurance and even, though not often, those who do not have health insurance (not to mention a co-pay).* This is still another reason health insurance is so expensive.

Here I want to say a few words about *underpaying* our nurses. Why should a licensed nurse practitioner that also makes diagnoses, decides on treatment and prescribes drugs, accept significantly less pay than the doctor she substitutes for? Registered nurses who actually carry out the prescribed treatments have equally responsible jobs, and deserve proportional compensation. Underpayment goes all the way down the medical hierarchy, with nurse assistants at the bottom (typically immigrants from Southeast Asia). If somebody is overpaid, it is medical management: no manager will ever be paid less than those he is in charge of!

Let me now turn to the malpractice insurance that doctors have to purchase. Dr. Atul Gawande, a distinguished surgeon and author of three bestselling books on medicine, writes, "Malpractice suits are a feared, often infuriating, and common event in a doctor's life...The average doctor in a high-risk practice like surgery or obstetrics is sued about every six years."[26]

There is not an hour on virtually any TV channel that malpractice lawyers do not advertise their services.† We do know that doctors have to pay enormous malpractice insurance premiums. We also know that in order to minimize the danger of being sued for malpractice, doctors practice what is called "defensive medicine:" they administer unnecessary tests and procedures.

How much do malpractice litigations – real and anticipated – can cost Americans? Although there have been quite a few studies on this issue, there

---

* For example, within the same hospital, charges for a coronary bypass may vary by a factor of three.
† In my essay *Litigation Explosion*
(www.SayNoToBoredom.com/Litigation_Explosion.html) I tell a story of how a 1977 Supreme Court decision unleashed the avalanche of litigations.

are still no reliable data. Hence contradictory information can be found on the Internet.

Based on a Gallup survey, a 2010 article on the site of American Orthopaedic Surgeons[27] claimed that 21% of doctors' practice was defensive, ordering some unnecessary extra 35% of diagnostic tests, 29% of lab tests, 19% of hospitalizations, and 8% of surgeries. Also, 14% of unnecessary prescriptions were issued in order to avoid lawsuits. As a result, as estimated by doctors, 34% of health care costs were attributed to defensive medicine.

If this is true, a reform (a so-called "tart reform") that would slash malpractice expenses and eliminate defensive medicine would significantly decrease our health care costs. But that would be an easy remedy, and sounds too good to be true.

Another (2011) estimate claims that the cost of defensive medicine reaches only 10% of total health care spending.

On the other hand, the article written by an all-star Harvard team[28] draws a different picture, though the authors note that the data on malpractice and defensive medicine costs are not highly reliable. They estimate defensive medicine costs at $45.59 billion in 2008, with hospitals' and physicians/clinical services' shares at $38.79 and $6.80 billion respectively. As for the indemnity payments, they are estimated to be only $5.72 billion, accompanied by administrative expenses of $4.13 billion, over half of which ($3.09 billion) are lawyers' fees. If those data are correct then the total cost of our medical liability system – $55.64 billion – was just 2.4% of the total health care spending in 2008.

From the numbers above one can see that a tort reform would not significantly decrease direct health care cost. There are, however, two important factors to consider.

The first is a moral factor. A study has shown that every year one third of all orthopedic surgeons, one third of all emergency physicians, and one third of all trauma surgeons are sued.[29] Many physicians, as well as the majority of resident doctors participating in the study "viewed every patient as a potential law suit." This is a powerful psychological factor, although, 70% of lawsuits are either dropped by the plaintiff or won by the doctors.[23] And yet, the threat is ever present.

Here is the second factor. Something important is missing from the above-mentioned estimates of the "direct" malpractice and defensive medicine costs. Malpractice insurance premiums that doctors pay are gigantic. They vary from state to state and differ for various specialties. The most "dangerous" professions are surgery and ob-gyn. A general surgeon pays premiums ranging from $30,000 to $300,000 a year. An obstetrician may pay 50% more.[26]

However, nobody knows how much all our doctors pay to the insurers. What is known is that malpractice insurance companies' profit margins range from 5.9 to 74.8%, with an average of 31.2%.[30] Doctors pay all that money from their earnings and after taxes. I am not sure that this huge amount has been accounted for in what is called "health care expenditure:" Is this the money spent on health care? Thus, although a reform that would slash malpractice premiums and indemnity payments would appear to have only a tiny effect on the "direct" health care cost, but to doctors it would provide significant relief. The increase in their income might trickle down to decreasing their bills.[*]

The government is planning to reduce payments to Medicare providers. This would be more acceptable to physicians if a tort reform slashed down the malpractice payments. But thus far a tart reform is only in the planning stages. It deserves a higher priority.[†]

A few words in defense of malpractice insurance. It is, obviously, a kind of *quality control* of the health care system. It may be less expensive (as in the other countries we have visited), but it is necessary. In some countries, the so-called "contingency fee" litigations ("pay if we win") are prohibited. However,

---

[*] Prof. Uwe Reinhardt in the interview I am quoting below said: "The AMA [American Medical Association] has estimated it could be up to 10 percent [of unneeded tests administered]; we don't really know what it is. I also tell doctors: 'Well, on the other hand, these tests are profitable for you. So if we abolished malpractice, would you give up 10 percent of your income?' And that's not so clear to me whether they wouldn't do these tests anyhow."

[†] There is good news. After this book has been finished, in 2015, in two states: Georgia and Florida a substitute for malpractice insurance was proposed (http://www.medscape.com/viewarticle/840337_print). If passed, the bills would bury the the the current medical tort system, in stead establishing "Patients' Compensation Systems." Let me quote from the source above. "...patient, via a patient advocate, would appeal to the system to investigate his or her injury. The full record would be reviewed by a rotating collection of medical experts in the relevant field. If this panel agreed that the injury was avoidable, the case would be referred to a compensation committee to make payment. ... Physicians would not need to purchase medical malpractice insurance, because they could not be sued. Instead, they would pay an annual contribution to administer the program. A family practitioner, for example, would pay $3900 per year; an orthopedic surgeon, $15,600 per year; and a spine surgeon, $17,500 per year. The specialists with the highest contribution rate, pediatric neurosurgeons, would pay $25,300 per year. These rates would be significantly below the current market rate for professional liability premiums—which typically cover only $1 million of liability." The lawyers would probably fight tooth and nail.

in the U.S., like in Canada, France, Japan, and U.K. they are allowed. In the U.S. it is a powerful stimulus to sue. How many people would hang up on a lawyer who suggests suing a doctor on the condition that the client pays if the lawsuit is successful? Actually, it looks like many Americans do hang up: "Of every one hundred Americans injured in an accident, only ten make a liability claim, and only two file a lawsuit."[31] However, as Princeton University Professor Uwe Reinhardt, an expert in health care policy and economics (whom I have already quoted), noted, [32]

> ...in countries where the lawyer has to get paid to do the work, and the losing party has to pay the party that prevailed their court costs, in such a system, low-income [plaintiffs] would never bring suit; they would never have a hope. So actually, as un-American as this may sound, I'm actually in favor of the present system until we have something better.

Having paid all business expenses and malpractice premiums, a doctor brings home what amounts to only a 10% share of total health care spending.[33] This confirms the second answer to the question of whether cutting doctors' incomes would save our health care system. The analysis shows[30] that even if doctors' incomes were slashed by 20% (which would be utterly impossible!) that would save only 2% of our health care costs.

Having discussed all the suspicious causes of our *money rotting*, I could not find THE single most important one.

Here are the major 2011 categories (as was reported in the January 2013 issue of Health Affairs):[*34]

Hospital Care	33.%
Physician and clinical services	21.%
Prescription drugs	10.%
Dental and other care[†]	20.%
Other professional services	7.%
Direct administrative costs[11]	13.%

The administrative cost is enormous, but the rest looks reasonable.

And yet, we do burn money, almost everywhere, across the board. Here is how:

The 2012 report issued by the Institute of Medicine of the National

---

[*] The numbers do not add up to 100%, because the last number is from a different source.

[†] The source does not explain what "other care" means.

Academies[35] claims that $750 billion, close to 30% of our total health care expenditure, is wasted annually.

Here is the breakdown: [36]

Unnecessary services:	7.8%
Ineffective care delivery	4.8%
Excess administrative cost	7.1%
Inflated prices	3.9%
Fraud	7.8%

I would like to return to the graph at the beginning of this chapter.

Comparing health care expenses of the U.S. and France, we saw that if the U.S. were as affluent as France, our health care expenses would be 1.4 times (France's *Affluence Factor*) less: $5,600 per capita rather than $7,800. This is shown on the graph as a circle above France's diamond: a fat circle on the

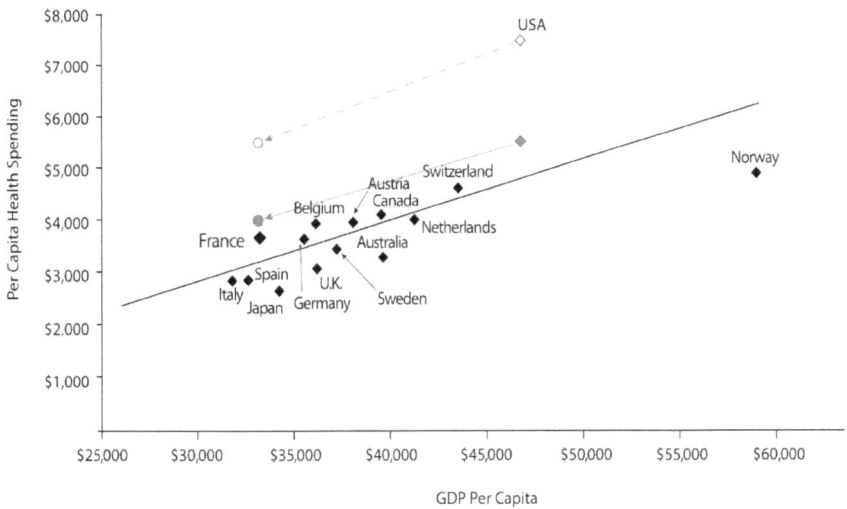

previous diagram or an unfilled circle on the diagram above. Now we know that almost 30% of our health care expenses – about $2,300 – are wasted, originating from various drawbacks in our system. Subtracting this amount from our expenses, we arrive at $5,500, shown as a new diamond on the diagram above (the unfilled diamond and the unfilled circle with a dotted arrow between correspond to "uncorrected" spending of the previous diagram). Were the U.S. in France's shoes: being less affluent by factor 1.4, our expenses would be almost exactly as those of France: only $4,000 (a fat circle above the France's diamond). Now, looking at the graph, we see that both the diamond and the circle: either the U.S. being "itself" or in France's shoes, fit well the "living according to one's means" straight line. Although the data I am analysing are from 2008, the picture is also valid today.

Now let us see what those wasted expenses are.

Unnecessary services: In most cases overuse by doctors and hospitals of sophisticated procedures, administering possibly unnecessary tests, and prescribing expensive drugs, are not only responses to our wish to be as healthy as we can be. The threat of malpractice is always looming over doctors no matter what they do. Administering unnecessary procedures is often part of defensive medicine. An interesting and multi-faceted example is cesarean section.

We hate pain and do not tolerate it well. Pharmaceutical companies supply us with a spectrum of drugs for pain of every variety. Giving birth to a baby is a painful process (remember: "In pain you will bring forth children," Genesis, 3:16) that can be avoided if the baby is safely delivered surgically, and the mother does not feel severe pain. (The pain in the post-surgery period is very much less severe than the pain experienced during the natural birth process.) Like any surgery, the cesarean section has its medical "do's and don'ts." On the other hand, under the possibility of complications, doctors will often recommend and even encourage cesarean sections, thus practically guaranteeing avoidance of a malpractice suit.

Ineffective care delivery is mostly caused by the fragmentation of our system. Too often there is no communication among the doctors involved in a patient's treatment and the patient, leading to duplication of efforts. Just two examples. A PCP sends a patient for an X-ray, and then refers him/her to an orthopedist, who repeats the test. A specialty doctor may not have access to the patient's blood test results administered by the PCP, and repeats the tests. Ineffectiveness also results from overuse of doctors and other personnel due to many factors; some of them I already discussed. The PPO system ("preferred provider organization") where a patient decides what specialty doctor should be visited, is another source of ineffective care delivery. I will be discussing this issue below.

Excess administrative cost: As we can see from the figures above, this is half of the total administrative cost. Not only is it an enormous bureaucracy composed of thousands of insurance companies. More important is that we do all documentation on paper--endless forms to be filled out by patients and doctors that are later transferred to computers. I have already discussed the "smart card" problem, which does not seem to be easily resolved. As for the insurance companies' bureaucracy, apparently we will have to live with it, with no light at the end of the tunnel...

Where Are We?

Inflation of prices is easily visible. The cost of new drugs and sophisticated high-tech tests and procedures (robotic surgeries are in the offing!) is growing. And the high-tech equipment and new drugs are more expensive in the U.S. than in other countries. In spite of that, both high-tech diagnostic services and procedures are more readily available in the U.S. than in other countries and are more often used. Companies manufacturing advanced equipment and drugs try to get the desired profit in the U.S. where, unlike other countries, the prices are not regulated. Some drug prices that Americans have to pay are exorbitant: for example, Novartis's Gleevec – a "Magic Cancer Bullet" to treat chronic myeloid leukemia – that may cost $100,000 per year. Americans are bombarded by TV ads for new and expensive drugs. In many cases the new drugs are no better than the existing ones, and the list of possible side effects that the advertisers must disclose is often frighteningly long. And yet, people ask their doctors to prescribe those drugs! Should not such ads be prohibited? (Our poor First Amendment!)

Of course, doctors and hospitals take advantage of our desire to spend more for treatment: hence the overuse of sophisticated and expensive procedures.

Just two examples.

America is a nation of back pain: we do not walk, we drive. Sitting for hours in a car or in front of TV is not good for our spine. If one is in pain, surgery seems to be a quick fix. Many orthopedists encourage people to have surgery. Ten years ago I agreed to it, although I rejected "fusion," a more radical and widely suggested surgery. For me the surgery was not a "fix," as it was not a fix for thousands of people who hoped for one. As a legacy of surgery I have a numb foot, but I can live with it. An alternative to back surgery is a conservative treatment based on physical therapy and enhanced physical activity in general. For me it has been yoga. Now my back is strong and I can do such strenuous things as splitting wood.

Another example is coronary bypass. It is often considered an unnecessary radical procedure, performed at the slightest suspicion of a heart attack, whereas in many situations change of lifestyle and conservative treatment would do the job without risk of complications and at significantly less cost. This example, however, invites controversy. When a heart attack is at issue, how can one be certain that an urgent measure can be postponed? Bypass and stent surgeries have saved thousands of lives.

There is also the sociological factor of overpaying for services: how people perceive those who are not healthy. Americans tend to hide their health problems from employers, employees, schoolteachers, and even friends – because "it isn't cool" to be sick and it's not nice to complain. As my friend's secretary used to say, "You should ALWAYS be happy. If you are not happy something's wrong with you!" But you cannot be happy if you have a heart condition or diabetes or depression. Americans are health conscious. Although they do not visit doctors as often as patients in the other countries we have visited, they are willing to pay more, even if procedures are not necessary, to try to remain healthy or recover faster, not because of a work ethic but so as not to lose their jobs.

Prevention failure: It seems to be more costly than the 2% listed above. If an illness has not been diagnosed in time, or misdiagnosed, its treatment becomes more expensive, sometimes *much* more expensive. Periodic prophylactic screening that would enable early diagnosis was not covered by many insurance policies before Obamacare. How efficient it will be under the new rules is to be seen.

Fraud: The major part of that enormous almost 8% waste is probably "institutionalized" fraud perpetrated by hospitals and doctors to overcharge those who have health insurance to cover losses for underpayment by those who do not. I already discussed this issue, and will discuss below Medicaid and Medicare fraud in detail.

Let me return to the issue, which, in my view, if resolved, could, reduce our health care expenses.

If one has PPO insurance (as well as Medicaid and Medicare), one may always see a specialist of one's choosing whenever one feels that this is just the specialist one needs to see. It actually means that the "self-diagnosis" is right and the choice of the specialty doctor is correct.

To come up with a correct diagnosis is a tedious and complicated process. A good diagnostician must first know how to listen to a patient. Everything the patient says may be important, even if the patient inadvertently shifts from the sickness to other topics. "Old school" doctors knew that making a diagnosis began with observing how a patient entered the doctor's office. Today, this stage of diagnosing has been eliminated: instead we sit (sometimes for a long time and sometimes dressed in only a paper gown) in a bare room with multiple diplomas and certificates on the walls waiting for the doctor to appear, possibly for just a few minutes.

Obviously, it is a doctor who should first hear one's complains and ascertain if he/she is able to put a diagnosis and administer treatment. And yet, the initial diagnosis is often left to the patient, who chooses a specialist he or she believes to be the right one. Not only is this an abuse that overburdens the system financially and overloads physicians. It may also have serious consequences for the patient's health because the specialist may not be the right one, and then the second may follow, etc.

If there is a *gate*, with a primary care physician as a "gatekeeper" (as in HMOs – Health Maintenance Organizations – and Medicare Advantage), the chance that a doctor's referral of the patient to an inappropriate specialist lessens. However, a gatekeeper may be biased and may attempt to minimize expenses or maximize income (e.g., not referring the patient to a specialist or a hospital even if it is medically necessary, but instead trying to take care of the issue at his/her office). As we saw, attempts in France to introduce gatekeeper control over referrals to specialists met active resistance. Even higher bills did not prevent the French from seeing whatever doctors they chose.

A gatekeeper system would probably slash the costs of our health care and decrease the unwitting abuse of the system. However, I would not insist on that: our HMOs have not been very popular.

Could *rationing* of health care be a solution? A significant chunk of what we spend on health care is spent to treat a small group of people: "In 2009, half of all health care spending was used to treat just 5% of the population."[37] Today people live longer: one of eight Americans is over 65 years old. This number will dramatically increase when baby-boomers begin entering that club en masse. Many of elderly have multiple chronic conditions requiring expensive treatment. And society would not condone sacrificing an 80-year-old human being by refusing a life-saving procedure that could extend that person's meaningful life. Rationing health care is a no-no in America, no matter how economically beneficial it could be. Being an elderly citizen who has recently overcome a complicated (and very expensive!) surgery,[*] I agree with most Americans.

However, the catch here is the word "meaningful." Would a late-stage cancer patient benefit from an experimental drug with yet unknown side effects, or would a hip replacement for an 82-year-old stroke survivor prolong his/her meaningful life? Even to "survive" intensive care after surgery may be questionable (chances may be as low 15-25%). Many more examples have to do with chemotherapy treatment during the last stages of cancer that may bring more suffering, but would not prolong life. Close to a quarter of all Medicare expenses are spent treating only five percent patients in their end-of-life stage.[38] The enormous resources are spent to prolong human suffering with the intension to prolong their lives.

It is not "rationing" that I am talking about. There is an area of health care

---

[*] First chapters of this book were written in a rehab center, with my MacBook unsteady on my knees!

called palliative care directed at relieving or preventing patients' suffering. Hospice care in the final stages of illness is a branch of it. Unfortunately, it is underused (for metastatic lung cancer – by 50%) in spite of the fact that it

> ...has enabled countless people worldwide to die with dignity. Through focusing on the patient rather than the disease, individuals can spend the last weeks of their lives in an environment where hospice caregivers minimize their pain, maximize their comfort, and provide bereavement services for loved ones and family members.[39]

This is because many patients (and their families) are in denial of inevitability of death in the situations of prolonged illness. And even if they know that death is imminent, they are unaware that there are other options of treatments that may enhance the quality of life, rather than degrade it as radical treatments inevitably do. Doctors, in their turn, often do not inform patients about those options.

One of the functions of "Death Panels"[40] – as conservatives call the *Independent Payment Advisory Board* of Obamacare – is to encourage doctors to discuss with patients optimal strategies of treatments in their last days of life. It is to begin with discussing with patients their *living wills* – their voluntary instructions to family and doctors regarding prolonging medical treatments – which, according to law (having nothing to do with Obamacare), every patient has to have (but many do not even know what it is!). On this stage of Obamacare nobody knows how these "Death panels" will function, but I do not see anything bad in helping people to achieve peace of mind after months of suffering, and spend the last days of their lives quietly preparing themselves for the end. Even if the main objective of explaining people how to get rid of pain and suffering is economic one, I do not see anything immoral in it.

As I already mentioned, what people pay for services is not the same for everybody. Medicaid people pay very little – virtually nothing, and Medicaid's payments to doctors are meager. Those eligible for Medicare pay monthly fees and are also responsible for co-payments and 20% of the bills.

The people outside these two categories either cannot afford insurance or manage to pay for it with or without the help of their employers. As I also mentioned, in order to survive, both doctors and hospitals *must* overcharge those who *are able* to pay. Insurance typically pays those bills, and this trickles down to everybody's insurance premiums, to which deductibles and co-payments also have to be added. This means that those who purchase private insurance are actually subsidizing through their taxes Medicaid and Medicare services, as well as emergency rooms and the hospital expenses unpaid by those who were unable to pay. That is one of the reasons insurance premiums are high and are unaffordable for millions of people.

Finishing the "overspending" topic, should I also mention greed as an unfortunate and powerful factor that costs our health care system dearly? Just think about surgeons deliberately encouraging patients to agree to procedures that are more dangerous or serious than necessary. As I have learned, in 2009 a group of five neurosurgeons

> performed the third-highest number of spine fusions in the country on Medicare patients. In addition to what Medicare paid them with tax dollars, the surgeons received $7 million directly from Medtronic, the company that makes the metal implants.[41]

Obviously, Medtronic has a program of awarding surgeons who use their devices: the five surgeons mentioned are just one example. And this is an operation, which, as I mentioned, is not effective; conservative treatment should be administered instead.

This is just one of many examples that can be found. The most ridiculous (if not disgusting!) in my view is paying huge salaries and bonuses to CEOs and higher management of non-profit hospitals. In the same book[38] (p. 130) the author references Kaiser Health Care News, 2011, claiming that in 2009 CEOs of three Children Hospitals (non profit!) in Kansas City, Missouri, Milwaukee, Wisconsin, and Akron, Ohio each received over $5 million as annual compensation. These nonprofit hospitals are not unique: huge salaries and bonuses not only for CEO's, but also for bureaucrats of lower level are typical today, with medical workforce squeezed to an almost impossible minimum. And hospitals barrage communities with requests for donations! Shall I (or we) stop giving to non-profit hospitals? Greed is deplorable no matter where it shows its ugly face. In health care it is especially shameful.

All the above being said, the main factor in our health care spending and individual expenses is the enormous cost of health care itself. An avalanche of new life-saving procedures, tests, and more efficient drugs is changing the face of medicine and health care. They are extremely expensive to develop and implement. If the growth proceeds as it has been going, then by 2035 health care costs may outgrow people's incomes.[42] Would radical health care reform do the trick? Let us hope so.

Now let me turn to other "somethings" that are rotting in our "kingdom." It is not "money rotting" because the issues I am going to discuss have either completely or partly fallen out of our health care. I would like to focus on three issues: "the maladies of our head," long-term health care (LTC) and maternity care.

Our Head

is the most important part of our body. Unlike a hip or a knee it cannot be replaced. There is also no head transplant. If you have lost your head, you are done.* Our head houses three outside organs: eyes, ears and teeth. It also houses the brain, which is our thinking vehicle.

Vision and hearing problems can be covered by one's insurance, although hearing aids and eyeglasses are not covered. And they are expensive. Medicare patients pay for them; Medicaid patients do not.

Dental care requires special insurance. Such insurance typically pays less than 50% of treatment costs. Everybody knows that installing a crown, a bridge or an implant can be a budgetary disaster. (Until recently, most insurance policies did not cover anything to do with implants.) Medicaid patients in Massachusetts do not have to pay for most dental work, (excluding implants). Again, the elderly, on Medicare, have to pay for dentist visits.

As for mental conditions, that is where our health care system fails miserably. Among the numerous maladies that our doctors treat, mental health issues are pariah.

Mental disorders are common everywhere: both around the world and in the U.S. According to the National Institute of Mental Disorders,[43] "An estimated 26.2 percent of Americans ages 18 and older — about one in four adults — suffer from a diagnosable mental disorder in a given year." The most widespread disorder – depression – afflicts one in 10 adults. If not treated properly and in a timely manner, depression can lead to suicide.† ("More than 90 percent of people who kill themselves have a diagnosable mental disorder, most commonly a depressive disorder or a substance abuse disorder"[40]). More serious disorders, like schizophrenia and bipolar disorder, afflict close to 7% of Americans, not to mention mood disorders, anxiety, panic disorders and others, which require physicians' or psychologists' interventions. The list is long. And according to a Harvard University study, 18% of people with psychiatric

---

* –"What is the name of that German guy I have lost my head over?" –"Alzheimer?"

† I already mentioned a high rate of suicides among doctors. "Physician suicide is medicine's darkest secret, and our code of silence is maintained by layers of lies", claims Pamela L. Wible, MD, who has managed to escape tragedy, in her article: *Physician Suicide 101: Secrets, Lies, and Solutions* (Medscape, Nov. 13, 2014): http://www.medscape.com/viewarticle/834434_5; Here are some lies attempting to cover the suicide: hanging – "asfixia;" substance overdose – "accidental overdose;" suicidal jump – "accidental fall;" gunshot wound – accidental shot, etc. "Physician suicide death certificates are miscoded by physicians even when there is clear evidence of suicide intent including a suicide note."

disorders commit at least one act of violence in a year.[44] *

For mental conditions there are special insurance codes[†] that signal insurance companies: "Do not pay!" or "Pay as little as possible." As I discuss in the next chapter based on the data from the table there, we have less psychiatric clinics and doctors than the other countries. This is not to mention that something is wrong with our attitude towards the mentally ill. Among the homeless people that we see on our streets, 20% to 25% need psychiatric care,[45] but they are neglected. It is sad…

Long-Term Care

Long-term care (LTC) is one of the most important health care issues in developed countries. The countries we have visited are more or less prepared (at least they are attempting to be prepared) for the invasion of the elderly. Societies are catastrophically aging, and the number of people over 65 increases dramatically. At this age even relatively healthy people become victims of a host of illnesses, Alzheimer's disease being the most threatening among them.

Initially Obamacare contained a provision related to LTC: the *Community Living Assistance Services and Support* (CLASS) Act originally introduced by Edward Kennedy. CLASS would authorize LTC care for all Americans, who would be automatically enrolled in the program.[46] In an October 15, 2011 letter to senior Democrats and Republicans in Congress, Secretary of Health and Human Services Kathleen Sebelius informed them that the CLASS program is not financially sustainable. But the bitter and shameful truth is that

> …it was easier for the Administration and vocal GOP critics of the program to kill CLASS than to answer the real question: How will the U.S. finance the long-term care needs of 20 million Americans who will need personal assistance within the next few decades?[47]

Why is the LTC issue so difficult to handle? Let me discuss briefly what the most threatening old-age sickness is and why it is so dangerous. What I mean is the so-called *dementia*, the gradual loss of memory and deterioration of other cognitive functions, as well as the ability to perform activities of daily living

---

* "Mass shootings" that has become frequent in schools and on college campuses is the issue that cannot be eliminated by tighter gun control, because most murderes were mentally unstable and needed psychiatric help.

† My friend was astonished to have found a $900 unpaid bill for a visit to a neurologist with his wife diagnosed with Alzheimer's. The explanation? The doctor accidentally gave a psychiatric code for dementia; otherwise Alzheimer's dementia – the abode of neurologists – would have been completely paid for.

(known in the literature as ADL). It has to do with degeneration of brain cells.

Dementia may be caused by a head trauma[*] or a tumor; such dementia can sometimes be reversed. More serious dementia is vascular; it is caused by strokes, even by repeated micro-strokes that may happen unnoticed. The most widely spread kind of dementia was discovered and first described by a German psychiatrist and neuropathologist Alois Alzheimer in 1906.[48]

Sixty to 80% of dementia patients die of Alzheimer's disease (AD). AD is, potentially, the most serious danger to be encountered by humankind.[49]

It is extremely difficult to distinguish between vascular and AD dementias, although doctors often declare AD as a diagnosis. However, upon autopsy, the difference is clearly seen: the brain cells of AD patients are immersed in a gray matter, a starch-like protein, called *beta-amyloid.*

Dementia is a sickness of the elderly.[†] It progresses with age: 5 to 8% of people are afflicted between ages 65 and 75; 15 to 20% between ages 75 and 85, and 25 to 50% over the age of 85. Only 1% of people with AD are afflicted with the disease because of some defects in their chromosomes. However, there is no way to separate out this group without a sophisticated genetic analysis. It is easier when AD is in the family and early onset of AD is observed through generations or siblings. Today 5.2 million Americans are diagnosed with AD. In the near future, when baby-boomers enter this dangerous age, the AD population will significantly increase. By 2050, between 11 and 16 million Americans will be diagnosed with AD. The total annual cost of supporting the afflicted will rise from $172 billion (in 2010) to $1.08 trillion in 2050.[50]

---

[*] "A study of former NFL players suggests that football players also may be at increased risk for mild cognitive impairment or similar cognitive decline, perhaps as a result of repeated head injury during the athletes' sports careers. In fact, 75 former professional football players are suing the NFL, alleging that the league concealed information about the harmful effects of concussions on the brain for decades." (http://www.cnn.com/2011/HEALTH/07/25/alzheimer.disease/index.html).
A growing number of reported concussions among children playing soccer may result in abandoning this popular game.
[†] I have come across a research paper that claims that we are facing an AD epidemic. The author notes that, before 1960 very little AD was mentioned in medical literature, although the illness had pronounced symptoms. Then only 2% of people at 85 had the disease, whereas today it is 50%. "This dramatic spike over 40 or so years, ... cannot be accounted for by an aging population." Here is the author's proof. As a sickness of old age, AD's incidence should have correlated with the number of femur or hip fractures. The latter increase with age proportionally, while the former increase exponentially, like AIDS. Of course, this is only a hypothesis (*Are We Experiencing an Alzheimer's Epidemic?*: http://www.medscape.com/ viewarticle/590106).

Where Are We?

And there is no cure.[*]

Some people believe that effective drugs exist and that AD is curable. However, currently accessible drugs may be effective only in the early stages of AD. But what is "an early stage"? There are no reliable "markers" for early diagnostics, and when AD symptoms become pronounced, it is possible that the illness began some 10 years earlier, with a large portion of the brain already conquered by *beta-amyloids*.

The 2011 *AD World Conference in Paris* identified some risk and prevention factors.[51] Based on a mathematical model, scientists estimated that three million people in the world could avoid acquiring AD if negative lifestyle factors were decreased only by 25%. In particular, they concluded that

> in the United States, physical inactivity had the biggest association with Alzheimer's out of the risk factors studied, followed by depression and smoking. Midlife hypertension, midlife obesity, low educational attainment and diabetes are other risk factors.

Some of this statement's claims do not seem to be true. Obesity, diabetes, depression, and smoking though contributing to AD are severe problems in their own right. Besides, smoking in America is less popular than in other countries (see the table). "Midlife obesity" is, in fact, one of the symptoms of decline in physical activity. And, as studies show, regular physical activity may be an important factor in postponing AD. As one can see from the table, the prevalence of dementia in America is more or less the same as in other countries where the above "causes" of dementia are less pronounced.

Educational level does seem to be an important factor. However, the onset of

---

[*] There is a coconut oil craze these days. The book by Bruce Fife, *the Coconut Oil Miracle* (Penguin Books, 1999; reprinted in 2000, 2002, 2004, and 2013) claims that coconut oil (CO) is an almost universal remedy, including for AD. There are also optimistic scientific papers. However, no rigorous double–blind study (neither a patient nor a doctor knows whether a true drug or a placebo is given to the patient) has been performed. A food supplement called Axona had an initial trial with optimistic results; however the manufacturer decided not to proceed with further trials, FDA approval, etc., and ruther threw Axone as a food supplement into market. An M.D. would say that, unless there is an FDA approval, she would not recommend CO as a "drug" for AD. However, someone diagnosed with cancer, tries whatever he (or some people) believes may help; the same with AD. If one has symptoms of dementia, one would try anything, even scientifically unproven. And this may be a right strategy. Besides, those with symptoms will not see a "scientifically approved " drug for at least a decade. As for now, there are anecdotal evidences that CO works. See, e.g., http://www.youtube.com/ watch_popup?v =ZZOR-Qd3QSg

---

175

dementia depends on how active one's brain cells are. Intensive intellectual activity, even in its most primitive form—solving crosswords or playing Sudoku—may postpone the onset of dementia. Learning and speaking foreign languages, and reading may also delay its onset. The best preventative is active creative work, no matter what kind.

Over 50 years ago the great Austrian psychologist and psychiatrist Viktor E. Frankl diagnosed a societal illness that had infected the entire developed world. It is the loss of meaning in the lives of millions of people. "Ever more people today have the means to live, but no meaning to live for." [*]

As for AD, a study has shown that "Higher levels of purpose in life reduce the deleterious effects of AD pathologic changes on cognition in advanced age."[52†] Another research confirms that those who have purpose and meaning in their lives are more resistant to cognitive impairment.

> ... results suggest that positive factors, such as having a sense of goal-directedness that guides behavior, may provide a buffer against negative health outcomes, particularly in old age. . . . Purpose in life is something we can actually modify in old age by giving older adults specific strategies they can use to find meaning in activities, achieve purposes, and goals. [53]

People in their 40s and 50s still have time to modify their lifestyle and decrease the potential risk of AD. Even retired people, who no longer have their everyday occupation, may find new purpose and meaning in their lives with an active social life, volunteering, study, or being involved with upbringing of their grandchildren. The personal computer is both our blessing and curse. It is a blessing because it opens up the whole world, inviting us to become part of the powerful development of life. It is a curse if its main purpose is to quell boredom. It cannot destroy it; rather it can only temporarily make it mute. It can also steal time that otherwise could have been spent in fitness centers and

---

[*] I discuss this issue in my book: *This Unbearable Boredom of Being. A Crisis of Meaning in America* (*iUniverse*, 2004), to which Dr. Frankl has written a preface.

[†] As for the kids (far away from AD), based on the research of prominent psychologists, I argue in my essay, *Does Life Have Purpose and Meaning? An Imaginary Conversation with Teenagers*
(http://www.saynotoboredom.com/Does_Life_Have_Purpose_and_Meaning.html) that if teenagers find nothing to devote themselves to while growing up, then it can be much more difficult for them to find a motivation that would make themselves fulfilled and happy later in life. (See, e.g. *The Development of Purpose During Adolescence*: http://web.stanford.edu/group/adolescence/cgi-bin/coa/sites/default/files/devofpurpose_0.pdf; *Spirituality Is Key To Kids' Happiness, Study Suggests:* http://www.sciencedaily.com/releases/2009/01/090108082904.htm.)

other meaningful activities.

Let me return to CLASS, the LTC program killed by the government before it was even born. It was supposed to be self-supporting and based on payroll deductions of participating workers, who would be automatically enrolled in it. The Congressional Budget Office (CBO) estimated that the deduction had to be on average $123 per month. More realistic estimates suggested much higher deductions, about $180–$240. The enrollees would have to contribute to the program for at least five years, only to receive shockingly small benefits: $55 to $75 daily (adjusted for inflation), or $20,000 to $27,000 annually.

How much care can be purchased for that money?[54] In the Boston area, the median costs are: for in-home care provided by an agency, $25/hr ($150 for a 6-hour day); for assisted living (single occupancy), $135/day ($4,000/month); and for a nursing home, $330/day ($120,450/year). Even the most "socialistic" health care systems that we visited were not covering the complete LTC cost. However, they did provide affordable supplemental insurance (and the nursing home costs there were significantly lower than in America).

One can also purchase LTC insurance in the U.S. For a 65-year-old the least expensive policy, covering $150/day for two years, adjusted for 4% inflation, would cost $158/month ($1,896/year, with the maximum spending of $109,500). This is a policy for which I would have been eligible as a government retiree if I were 65. Now that I am fifteen years older, I would have to pay $309/month ($3,700/year) for the same policy, which would cover my nursing home stay for only two years. A larger coverage and for a longer term would obviously be more expensive.

This is a more or less typical LTC insurance policy. If it comes to a nursing home, with its close to $400/day cost, it would cover only some 40% of the cost, $54,000 a year, leaving almost $100,000 a year to be paid from my savings. After two years, I would be on my own, paying close to $150,000 a year possibly for a few more years.

Almost 10 years ago, when my wife and I were 70, we attempted to purchase a supplemental LTC insurance. We decided to purchase a better (than the one I mentioned) insurance plan. However, we did not pass a test for our eligibility for the preference rate because we were involved in a "dangerous activity": we scuba-dived and skied. As a result, we would have had to pay close to $6,000/year for the two of us. We refused. At that time I still believed that a comprehensive LTC reform was in sight. I do not believe that any more. And I hate to think of the day (G-d forbid!) when my family will completely exhaust our savings and succumb to welfare.

Our whole system of LTC financing is faulty, if not criminally faulty. A typical strategy that people use (and books have been written on how to do that best; see, e.g.,[55]) is the following: (1) One has to hide one's assets (by, for example, transferring them to one's children's accounts). (2) One should be careful, because the government will do a five-year back check. (3) One nevertheless has to have enough money to pay for two years in a nursing home. After that, having exhausted all assets, one becomes eligible for Medicaid and has a free ride for as long as one stays in a nursing home, which can be 3 to 8 years. If one has hidden all assets and does not have money to pay for at least a couple of years, it may be difficult to find a good nursing home, because nursing homes do not like Medicaid patients. On average, Medicaid pays for about 60% of nursing home residents and covers about half of the nursing home expenses. Is not it natural, that, as a result, 40% residents who have to pay the other half of these expenses are charged enormous amounts: $300–500/day? This situation is exactly the same as the overcharging by doctors and hospitals of those who carry health insurance.

The research undertaken by the Consumer's Union (Consumer Report, Oct. 1997) found that

> Only about 10 to 20 percent of elderly can afford long-term-care insurance . . . A tax deduction that few are likely to use or benefit from is not a rational approach to the problem of long-term care. That leaves Medicaid . . . Medicaid pauperizes the families who must use it, and encourages the non-poor to shelter assets to qualify. Older Americans shouldn't have to become experts in techniques for divesting themselves of assets in order to plan for long-term care. Nor should they have to rely on welfare to pay for it. Rather than saddle the middle class with expensive insurance costs for policies that may be inadequate and unavailable to sick people, the public deserves system like Medicare for long-term care. [*]

---

[*] I copied the following quote from my essay, "Long-Term Care:The LoomingCrisis"(http://www.saynotoboredom.com/longterm_care_The_Looming_Crisis.html) written over ten years ago. The essay was motivated by my discovery of the CBO estimates of the projected LTC costs and the total tax revenue for the period 2010–2030. I was astonished to learn that the LTC cost could be completely covered from taxes if the total tax revenue increased by just 5- 6%. As an example, I calculated that in the year 2000 a family with two dependents and the adjusted gross income of $50,000 would have paid only an additional $500 in taxes to contribute to the complete support not only of their parents or grandparents, but of all American elderly needing long-term care. I wrote a letter to the *Boston Globe* and two letters (with a few months' interval) to Edward Kennedy, without receiving even a thank you note in response. It would have been an easy solution, though impossible in today's America. Now I understand how naïve I have been.

So, now even the meager CLASS is dead. CLASS had to be self-supporting, financed only by enrollees' contributions such as Social Security, without any spending from the federal budget. At the same time Medicaid's and CHIP's projected spending between the years 2012 and 2022 would be $931 billion.[56] This says a lot about our government's spending priorities. Now that even a tiny hope for a meaningful LTC reform has disappeared America is silent. It is especially distressful that in no way will Medicaid be able to support the significant number of baby-boomers who will need LTC outside of their homes. It's dreadful even to think about it!

Returning to AD as the most important issue in LTC: In January 2011, President Obama signed into law the National Alzheimer's Project Act.[57] An *Advisory Council on Alzheimer's Research, Care, and Services* composed of 27 experts (15 of them government bureaucrats) will supervise development of the project. In May 2012, Health and Human Services Secretary Kathleen Sibelius, in a press release, outlined the National Plan to Address Alzheimer's Disease that was called for in the above-mentioned act.[58]

> To help accelerate this urgent work, the President's proposed FY 2013 budget provides a $100 million increase for efforts to combat Alzheimer's disease. These funds will support additional research ($80 million), improve public awareness of the disease ($4.2 million), support provider education programs ($4.0 million), invest in caregiver support ($10.5 million), and improve data collection ($1.3 million).

Through the National Institute of Health (NIH) our budget allocated in 2013 for Alzheimer's research $504 million. For 2014 and 2015 financing is projected to be $566 million.[59] Additionally, in April, 2013, The National Institute of Health (NIH) launched a ten year BRAIN (Brain Research Through Advancing Innovative Neurotechnologies) Initiative "to revolutionize the understanding of the human brain"[60] In 2015 BRAIN's budget will be $200 million.

Thousands of scientists are involved in AD research throughout the world. Both in the U.S. and in other countries the research goes in many directions. The unplowed field is tremendous. To begin with, we still do not know whether *beta-amyloid* that accumulates in brain cells is a cause of the disease or its consequence.* A promising direction of research is the development of an anti-Alzheimer's vaccine.

To be realistic: no society can support tens of millions of people in various stages of intellectual and physical deterioration. The most that can be done is

---

*Sometimes autopsies show that there are people whose brains were invaded by beta-amyloid who did not have any AD symptoms.

to provide financing for in-home services. This is what the countries we have visited have been aiming for: avoiding a nursing home for as long as possible. And yet, in my view, the only hope for our civilization is development of reliable and efficient anti-dementia drugs within 5-10 years. Thus far there was no solid ground for optimism.

Discussing LTC, I focused only on the care of people with dementia and AD. However, LTC has another function, End of Life Care (ELC): care for people terminally ill, even without AD symptoms. A National Academy of Science's Panel concluded that our system for handling end-of-life care "is largely broken and should be overhauled at almost every level."[61] The ELC system is extremely expensive because it provides patients with care and medicine that not only may not decrease their suffering, but even increase it. Above I mentioned palliative care, which begins with a thoughtful discussion among the patient's relatives and physicians concerning the best way to make the last period of the patient's life more comfortable and pain-free. Some insurance companies already pay for such discussions. Medicare should do likewise. There is no other way to make ELC efficient and less expensive without palliative care and cooperation with physicians. To create an efficient and viable ELC system is another of America's challenges.[*]

Maternity Care

The United States is the only democratic country that does not have *guaranteed* paid maternity leave.[62,63] All over the world, not only in Europe, but also in Africa, South America, and the Pacific, there are almost no countries that do not provide their pregnant women with at least partly paid maternity leave.

The Human Rights Watch, a New-York-based organization that usually focuses on violation of human rights in other countries (especially Israel but never in world dictatorships!), issued a critical report on work/family policy in the U.S. in November 2011 called *Failing its Family*. They claim that 178 countries in the world guarantee paid maternity leave, and over 50 countries also provide paid leave for new fathers. As for the U.S., it is in the company with Swaziland and Papua New Guinea.[64] Here is a partial list of countries that provide maternity leave (the six countries we have visited are in *italic*):[65]

Fully paid maternity leave: Argentina, 90 days; Chile 18 weeks; China 90 days; Egypt 90 days; *France 16 weeks*; *Germany 12 weeks*; India 12 weeks;

---

[*] The excellent book by Athul Gawande *Being Mortal. Medicine and What Matters in the End* (Metropolitan Books. Henry Holt and Company, New York 2014) discusses the endo-of-life in all facets.

Where Are We?

Israel 14 weeks; *Japan 14 weeks*; Malawi 8 weeks; Mexico 12 weeks; Morocco 14 weeks.

Partly paid maternity leave: Australia 12 weeks; Botswana 12 weeks; *Canada 50 weeks*; Czech Republic 28 weeks; Finland 105 days; *Great Britain 52 weeks*; Myanmar 12 weeks; New Zealand 14 weeks; South Africa 16 weeks.

Unpaid maternity leave: Papua New Guinea 12 weeks; Sudan 8 weeks; Swaziland 12 weeks; Zambia 12 weeks.

It is not wholly true that the U.S. is in the same category as undeveloped countries. It is true in that we do not have a *federal law* that *guarantees* parental leave on par with developed countries. What we have is the 1993 *Family and Medical Leave Act* (FMLA). For working women the act guarantees 12 weeks of unpaid leave but only if the company has more than 50 workers. Implementation of the law by different states is different.[66] Although about 60% of working women are covered by FMLA-related leave, only about one-fourth of U.S. employers offer fully paid "maternity-related leave" of various durations, and one-fifth of U.S. employers offer no maternity-related leave of any kind, paid or unpaid.[67]

Actually, parental leave that is authorized outside FMLA is much better. California, Hawaii, New Jersey, New York, and Puerto Rico have their own *Temporary Disability Insurance* that also applies to pregnant women. This insurance, however, does not guarantee job protection. California, New Jersey, and Washington have also passed *Paid Family Leave Acts* that cover pregnancy and also care for sick family members. Here is a listing of the benefits provided by both laws as of 2013:[68]

California:	6 weeks; 55 % – 60% of highest quarterly income, up to $1067
Hawaii:	26 weeks; 58% of average weekly wages, up to $535
New Jersey:	12 weeks; 66% of average weekly wages up to $584
New York:	12 weeks; 50% of average weekly wages, up to $170
Rhode Island:	30 weeks; 4.62% of the highest quarter wages, up to $736 plus 10% or 7% of weekly benefit for each of up to 5 dependents
Washington:	5 weeks: flat benefit $250/week (2009)
Puerto Rico:	26 weeks; 65% o of average weekly wages, up to $113

Other states are considering passing California-style maternity laws but the situation is not improving nationwide. The *Families and Work Institute* reported in 2008 that only 16% of companies with 100 or more employees provided fully paid maternity leave. In 1998 it was 27%.

Who Cares about Health Care?

In March 2009, President Obama created the *White House Council on Women and Girls*,[69] one of its priorities being evaluation and development of "policies that establish a balance between work and family." A new council... Come to think of it: what are those policies supposed to be? How can a "balance between work and family" be established? Is not that a prerogative of the family, and should not government have anything to do with it? American women do not need another council; they need comprehensive legislation.

By 2014 when Obamacare is fully implemented, new small and individual group insurance plans will have maternity leave among their benefits. Meanwhile, approximately 2.4 million women gave birth in 2012, and only 8% of those working in the private sector got maternity benefits.[70]

Based on interviews with dozens of parents, the *Human Rights Watch's* report that I mentioned above claimed that because of lack of paid leave, mothers often pay a heavy price by sacrificing their babies' health and their own. Numerous complications can occur even in the baby's anatomy.

Reading about our paternity situation will distress many readers, if not depress them. Come to think of it: When a woman carries her baby there is a man involved who will soon call himself father. He says he loves the baby's mother. But if he does, how is it possible that he allows her to drive to her workplace and work for eight hours a day till almost the very moment of birth, and then return to work as soon as she is physically able?

We are the richest nation in the world!* Do we know the numbers? Do we know how many miscarriages or birth complications occur because a woman has to work during the last week of her pregnancy? Two weeks? A month? Two months? And then go to work as soon as she is physically able to drive!

Why here, in the U.S., do we not hear serious discussion of this important issue? Why do men not insist, when they elect their congressmen and senators, that a maternity leave law be part of the platform of the would-be legislators? Even if the men who care for their pregnant working wives comprise only, say, 20 to 30% of married men, there would still be millions of them—a strong political force. Yet this is not a political issue. Those who vote – both for Republicans or Democrats – have wives who expect children. Don't they understand that it is simply inhumane and irresponsible in the 21st century to endanger the lives of their as yet unborn children and their wives by forcing them—their loved ones—to work till the very last day? My brain refuses to comprehend that.

---

* In India employers are *prohibited* from allowing women to work within six weeks after giving birth.

We have high infant mortality. In the next chapter I will attempt to partly exonerate our health care system from complete responsibility for that. Here, however, I want to discuss where we in fact are guilty.

The social causes of infant mortality, such as smoking, alcohol and drug use, poor nutrition, absent fathers, poverty, domestic violence, and so on exist in all countries, especially among people of low income and education, minorities among them. A health care system as such may not be responsible for those factors. However, such causes of infant mortality as inadequate funding and capability of perinatal health care, and insufficient public awareness of the problem can be blamed on the health care system.

In all the countries we have visited the latter factors are rarely involved. In France and Germany, for instance, high birth rate and survivability of babies is a serious social issue, and children's health is a high priority concern.

In the U.S. all the causes mentioned above may be blamed for higher infant mortality. As I mentioned, part of the responsibility also lies in in the fact that we as a nation do not care for expectant mothers. There are no statistics telling us how many children die prematurely because their mothers have to work till the very last day before giving birth.

Another factor may contribute to child mortality. If you look in the table at the data on the percentage of vaccinated children at age two, you will see that we are behind the other nations. The U.S. Centers for Disease Control and Prevention has formulated vaccination schedules for children ages 0 – 18.[71] However there is no federal law mandating vaccination.

State laws mandate vaccination for children entering school. However, all states allow exemption on medical grounds, 48 states – for religious reasons and 19 states for philosophical or other personal reasons. An unvaccinated child presents a danger not only to himself/herself but to others, especially to younger children whose immune systems may be weak.[72]

Because toddler vaccination is not mandatory, increasing numbers of parents refuse to vaccinate their children for fear of possible complications. These fears are based on popular myths about the dangers of vaccination.[73]

Virtually all drugs have side effects; vaccines are no exception. On average, every year about 100 million vaccinations are given, and there are only 90 or so childhood deaths that might or might not have been caused by the vaccination. The chance of contracting encephalitis from the vaccine is one in a million, whereas an unvaccinated child has a one in 1000 chance of suffering encephalitis as a complication of measles.

Although only about 2% of parents completely refuse to vaccinate their children, 1 in 10 skip at least some vaccinations. The statistics is blunt: in order to prevent the spread of serious diseases, 85 to 95% of the population needs to be vaccinated![74] Refusal to vaccinate children has dangerous consequences: some illnesses that were believed to have been eradicated (among them whooping cough, measles, mumps, meningococcal meningitis, encephalitis, and others) are experiencing resurgence.

This is a serious issue, which, again, is closely related to the drawbacks of our educational system that primarily teaches skills but neglects to provide people with solid knowledge including that about life science and medicine.

Medicaid and Medicare

Before I finish this chapter, I would like to return to our two government programs-- Medicaid and Medicare—which are also rotting in their own ways.

Both Medicaid and Medicare were created by the Social Security Administration in 1965.[75,76] These are two completely different programs, although people often confuse them. Let me begin with

Medicaid

This program was created in order to provide health care to people and families with low incomes, as well as to some people with disabilities, and the homeless. Only U.S. citizens and legal permanent residents are eligible. Medicaid is administered by each state and monitored by the federal government, which establishes requirements for service delivery, quality, funding, and eligibility standards. The program is jointly financed by states and the federal government (on average, the federal government covers 57% of expenses).

In 2012, the government's budget ($3.7 trillion) comprised some 23% of the GDP ($15.6 trillion). For health care, the budget reallocated 21.% (780 billion),[77] which equals about 5% of the GDP (not to be confused with the total 17.7% of health care expenses in the GDP). The government completely finances the Children's Health Insurance Program (CHIP), and Veteran Administration.

Before the June 27, 2012, Supreme Court ruling, Obamacare would have extended the Medicaid eligibility income to 138% of the federal poverty level (FPL).[78] In 2012, 54 million people were enrolled in Medicaid and CHIP.[79] Starting in 2014, the enrollment would increase, adding between 16 and 24 million people by 2019.[80] By that year the total Medicaid enrollment would comprise close to 25% of the population.

The situation dramatically changed after the Supreme Court ruling. The "forceful" expansion of Medicaid was found unconstitutional in that the federal government was prohibited from forcing states to accept new enrollees, and punishing those who would not by cutting government financing. As a result, Medicaid enrollment will not rise so dramatically pushing those who are ineligible to heavily government subsidized private insurance policies through *Exchanges*.

The states that agree to expand Medicaid enrollment will receive 100% federal financing through the years 2014-2016, decreasing to 90% by the year 2020. In 2013 and 2014 the rate of payment for Medicaid services will be raised to match Medicare payments, which are higher. The federal government will completely reimburse states for those expenses. States will also have to enforce the eligibility of children for Medicaid and CHIP and extend the funding through 2015. As of June 2013 at least thirteen states refused to expand Medicaid.

In order to better understand the financial structure of Medicaid, I present here a few federal guidelines (I am quoting from[81,82]):

> •Premiums remain prohibited for most children and adults below 150% FPL. (All *new* Medicaid enrollees below 138% FPL will not be paying any premiums
> either.) Most children and adults with income above 150% FPL, will now pay premiums, as well as cost-sharing of
> up to 20% of the cost of the service.
> •FY 2013 Maximum Nominal Copayment Amounts, depending on the state's cost of services between $10 and $50 (and over), varied from $0.65 to $3.90. Copayment for drugs (up to 150% FPL) was $3.80.
> •FY 2013 Maximum Nominal Deductible and Managed Care amounts were respectively $2.65 and $3.90.
> • FY 2013 non-emergency use of ER for enrollees up to 100% FPL was $3.90; for those of 101-150%FPL: $7.80.
> •Copayments cannot be imposed on emergencies, family planning, pregnancy-related services, and preventive services for children.
> •For some enrollee groups above 100% FPL, states may impose alternative out-of-pocket costs, which cannot exceed 5% of family income.

We see that the suggested cost sharing is minuscule[*]. Because Medicaid eats up the largest chunk of states' budgets (close to a quarter), some states attempt to

---

[*] I was unable to find a simple number: what percentage of Medicaid financing is covered by the beneficiaries. As if it were a national security secret...

increase the load on the enrollees. These attempts meet severe resistance.* The argument is that if the co-pay is too high, patients will not go to physicians; instead they will go to emergency rooms with more complicated health issues, thus increasing the load on the "non-poor." However, some states cannot survive fiscally without increasing Medicaid's fees.

An example: In 2010 Arizona increased co-pays for childless adults: for office visits – from $1 to $3; for non-emergency ER visits – from $5 to $30; the generic drug co-pay would be $4. (If a generic drug is unavailable, a brand name drug will cost $10.) In 2011 the Department of Health and Human Services approved these changes. Nevertheless, in its decision, the U.S. Ninth Circuit Court of Appeals rejected the co-pay charges imposed by the state.

Medicaid's budget is skewed: although 75% of its beneficiaries are adults and children, their benefits take only 30% of the budget, while the rest of the money is spent for the elderly and disabled, who comprise only 25% of the enrollees.

At the same time, the services for Medicaid elderly who are also enrolled in Medicare (the so-called dual-eligible) are first paid by Medicare; the rest is picked up by Medicaid. And the Medicaid elderly do not pay monthly Medicare fees. As we can see, Medicaid's budget is significantly eased while Medicare's is overloaded. Although the Supreme Court has had its say, the future of Medicaid is still in clouds...

Now I would like to discuss in more detail

Medicare

–the program that provides health care for the elderly – from 65 years old on – on which tens of millions of the elderly depend. Originally, Medicare consisted of two parts: Part A – hospital insurance, and Part B – medical insurance, covering doctor visits, tests, etc. Parts C (the so called "Medicare Advantage" plans), and D (prescription drug plans) were established respectively in 1997 and 2006.

In 2012, close to 60 million elderly were enrolled in Medicare. Millions upon millions of baby boomers will join it soon. By 2030, enrollment may reach 80 million! [83] The total cost of sustaining Medicare (including beneficiaries' monthly payments) will rise significantly from 3.6% of the GDP in 2012 to 5.6% by 2035. By 2087 it may reach 6.5%.[84]

As of 2013, all working Americans, irrespective of their age, pay the social

---

* Remember the "mini-revolution" in France in response to imposing a 1 Euro ($1.3) surcharge on all medical services?

security tax of 7.65%, known as FICA (after the Federal Insurance Contribution Act). Of that amount 6.2% covers social security benefits payable upon reaching retirement age, and 1.45% (raised in 2013 to 2.35% for incomes above $200,000) is the Medicare tax (HI–Hospital insurance) that pays for Medicare part A: hospital stay. Employers also pay the same fractions of the employees' salaries. The "social security" wages have a ceiling: $117,000, as of 2014. From the remaining salary, no matter how large, the 6.2% tax is not withheld. The Medicare tax is withheld from the total salary.[85]

Thus, while working, an American accumulates a significant amount of money, which will be used for his/her hospital care after the age of 65. Then, there will be no monthly payments, although one will have to pay $1,216 deductible. After that staying in a hospital for 60 days will be free; for the next 30 days one will have to pay $304, and in the next two months (up to the total of 150 days) – $608/day.

Having enrolled in Medicare part A, an American is also eligible to join Medicare part B – general medical insurance. Medicare B enrollment is mandatory unless one is covered by any other health insurance either through work or through a spouse. Medicare B is not free. Monthly payments depend on income and vary (for a single) from $104.9 for income $85,000 or less, to $335.70 for income over $213.000.[86] There is also a deductible of $147/ year.

Medicare A's expenses are almost completely (by 84%) paid from the FICA Medicare Tax, even though there are no monthly payments (although there is deductible and co-insurance). As for Medicare B, 74% of its cost is paid from general taxation accounted for in the federal budget, while the rest is covered by the elderly's monthly payments.[87] Medicare, like Medicaid, is called "entitlement." In my view, this is not quite fair: the elderly do pay from their own pockets a significant chunk of Medicare A's, and a quarter of Medicaid B's expenses.

Medicare B pays for a wide range of doctors' services, tests, and procedures. It establishes its own tariffs for every procedure and imposes these tariffs on providers. A doctor who agrees to work with Medicare also agrees to accept payments according to those tariffs, no matter how big the actual bill that a patient is expected to pay is. Of this approved amount, Medicare pays 80%. The remaining 20% is the responsibility of the patient and must be paid either out of pocket or through a supplemental insurance. There are also co-pays at the time of doctor visits.

Medicare parts A and B are called "traditional Medicare." Lately, supplemental programs have become popular. Among them is Medicare part D – prescription drug coverage, which is available through private companies.

The government pays (from general taxation) 83% of the cost, leaving the rest to the participants. The program is complicated and far from perfect. However, it is the only available program that eases the burden of paying market price for drugs. In 2012, about 23 million Americans were enrolled in Medicare D.[88]

The Medicare Advantage plan (sometimes called Medicare C) is a combination of Medicare B and private coverage. Those enrolled do not have to worry about paying the 20% unpaid by Medicare B. The Advantage plan completely pays the Medicare-approved bills. The patient is charged additional premiums as well as co-pays at the time of doctor visits. In 2012, more than 13 million Americans (27% of all beneficiaries) were enrolled in Medicare Advantage.[83]

Time and again we hear that Medicaid and Medicare are infested with fraud and abuse. Fraud is a problem of law enforcement. Only extremely severe deterrence (for which our society is not prepared) would be capable of eradicating fraud (and not only in Medicaid and Medicare).[*]

Increasing prison sentences and fines could at least keep fraud under some control. As for abuse, it is not always a criminal offense. Some people who might be accused of abusing Medicaid or Medicare are often unaware that they have abused the systems.

Many Americans do need health care subsidies. However, as we saw in other countries, if coverage is 100% and cost sharing is insignificant, abuse is inevitable. As I see it, abuse is an implicit ingredient of Medicaid, especially when a patient chooses to see a specialist when a visit to an internist would suffice. This is the opposite of the view that even an insignificant co-pay would discourage patients from seeing doctors.

---

[*] This actually touches on a more general issue. Our jurisprudence (and that of all democracies) is based on the concept of PUNISHMENT, hence the principle that punishment should not be too cruel and "disproportional." The concept of DETERRENCE is completely different: a possible punishment that would be capable of stopping crime MUST be "disproportional." We do know that the death sentence does not reduce "crimes of passion." However, it could completely eliminate white-collar crime, such as identity theft, embezzlement, or computer crimes such as hacking or spreading viruses. Imagine, death sentence without right of appeal for a *proven* identity theft. It is possible that only the very first sentenced person would be executed. There would be no more such crimes if a potential criminal knew that no life sentence or parole would save him. By the way, in the Old Testament G-d's death sentences for many "crimes" that would not even be considered as such today, are but DETERRENCE. Nine times in Deuteronomy, after imposing death as a punishment, the same words are repeated: "So you shall burn away what is bad from among you." Deterrence is allows *burning away* crimes. And G-d's cruel punishments in the Old Testament are but the very first use of DETERRENCE to insure social stability.

A few words about Medicaid fraud. "Organized fraud," where physicians in collaboration with criminals are involved in billing for nonexistent procedures, prescribing unnecessary drugs, etc., is a branch of organized crime and can be dealt with only by ruthless law enforcement measures. "Individual fraud" is different, and it can be stopped by proper deterrence. Here is a typical case: a patient sells his/her Medicaid card to a crook and then reports its loss, or receives a pain-killer prescription from a doctor under the false pretense of pain, and then sells the drug on the street. If people knew that such a kind of Medicaid abuse if caught would have them to pay a significant fine, lose Medicaid enrollment or go to jail, that would be enough to significantly curb this kind of abuse. But the warnings have to be strongly implanted in people's consciousness. However, I have not heard anything about such measures.

Like Medicaid, Medicare is not immune to fraud. However, most often fraud is perpetrated by hospitals and doctors' offices with the intent to overcharge Medicare patients, especially if a patient has supplemental insurance that will pay the bill anyway. Medicare will not pay for a procedure above its tariff; however, charging for services that were not rendered or procedures that were not performed, or "up-coding" the service (like charging for a surgery when only a bandage was applied) are typical abuses. In an ambulance bill one may often see a charge for the use of oxygen, though the condition did not require it and it was not used. At least a part of such fraud, though criminal, is "necessary" for providers as a remedy for Medicaid's and Medicare's underpayment. I discussed this situation above. There is also "truly criminal" fraud such as sending fraudulent claims by doctors, connected with organized crime. This is a serious crime to be investigated by the FBI.

As a government program, Medicare has some ugly features. Here is one of them.

A shocking example of ... may I call it an institutionalized fraud. This is a true story told by the *Boston Globe*.[89]. An elderly man was taken to a famous Boston hospital in a life-threatening condition after complications following surgery and stayed there for 10 days. "Nurses provided around-the-clock treatment, changing the 91-year-old's catheter, for example, and pumping him with intravenous drugs for suspected pneumonia." However, the hospital decided that the patient was not sick enough to qualify as an official "inpatient." For those 10 days that he was kept in the hospital "for observation," e.g., as an "outpatient," the total bill was $7,859. If he had stayed in the hospital as an inpatient, he would probably not have paid anything. Why? Medicare pays hospitals for inpatients more than for outpatients. However, Medicare punishes hospitals, accusing them of keeping patients when they could be quickly treated and sent home. "Observations" should last from 24 to 48 hours. But hospitals prefer, when possible, not to admit sick people as full-fledged inpatients in order to avoid punishment from Medicare for "improperly admitting patients." (About 8% of Medicare recipients stayed in hospitals as outpatients for longer than 48 hours in 2011, up from 3% in 2006.) Another factor: Hospitals are punished for re-admitting patients, which often happens with the elderly. So, hospitals are between Scylla and Charybdis.

As for Medicare abuse, in most cases it is unwitting; for example, seeing a physician for a very minor problem, even though the visit is not free. However, often, the elderly may be excused for being too cautious about their health.

In today's heated discussions of Medicare reform both the liberals and the conservatives agree that "Medicare as we know it" cannot exist any more. How can Medicare costs be decreased?

Republicans suggest a partial "privatization" of Medicare, which will allow beneficiaries either to stay with the old (but modified) Medicare, or use government grants that would allow them to purchase policies from private insurers. It is believed that competition among insurance providers will improve quality of care and make Medicare less costly.

Some of the proposals are raising the Medicare age to 67, raising the Medicare payroll tax, raising Medicare premiums for higher-income people, and adding co-payments to some services.

Obamacare hopes that the system can be restructured if the newly created panel of fifteen bureaucrats, the *Independent Payment Advisory Board* can cut spending. It is expected that its first significant action will be cutting Medicare fees to providers. When talking about making Medicare "less costly," both the liberals and the conservatives want to slash *government's* spending in order to decrease the budget deficit. Because it is unlikely that any such measures will decrease health care's *true cost*, it is the elderly who will have to pick up the tab.

To resume: Right now it is not clear what the Medicare's future will be.

And yet, come to think of it...When we talk about "Medicare's crisis," we mostly mean Medicare B. (Medicare A almost completely – by 84% – pays for hospital services from the money accumulated from the FICA tax and co-payments.) The financial crisis exists because the money the elderly pay monthly (plus co-pays) is insufficient. As I mentioned, it covers only some 25% of the cost of care for elderly people. The government has to cover the 75% balance of Medicare B expenses, and soon it will be unable to do that.

For reasons I do not understand, the two Medicare programs: A and B created in 1965 were treated differently since their inception. It had been decided that all working people had to have a kind of "savings plan" for paying hospital costs in later years and that was good. Why was there no similar savings plan created for paying for doctors' services in old age? And why don't we correct that mistake today?

Why not add to the 1.45% (or 2.35%) FICA Hospital Tax another tax that would allow an American to accumulate a significant amount of money to cover Medicare B expenses during his or her working life? Please bear in mind that I am not suggesting a new tax to cover "health care for all:" that is out of the question, and I am not that naïve to suggest it today. I am talking about an additional "pension plan." One would have to pay for covering one's own health care expenses decades later, being old and possibly infirm. It is quite possible that Medicare would then be sustainable. However, new taxes in today's political climate are anathema, and therefore my humble suggestion will not be heard. Such a shame...

Medicare for All?

Canada's Medicare is a Medicare for *all*, simply because it is their health care system. In America, it is also the object of all possible accusations, most of them false. However, we do tolerate Medicare for the elderly. Is Medicare for *all* possible in the U.S.?

Why not? Medicare has been good for the American elderly. It is their shield against the uncertainties of the private insurance market. As I mention in the concluding chapter, although the life expectancy at birth in America is lower than that in the other countries we have visited, the life expectancy for those over 65 is on par with the others. This is definitely because Medicare takes good care of the elderly.[*]

Unfortunately, President Obama has not taken the Medicare system as a blueprint for his "health care for all" reform. The main reason is obvious: Medicare is a single payer system, a "public option": everybody automatically participates in it and pays through payroll deductions and taxation. There are no personal insurance policies: everybody's money pays for everybody's health care. As I discussed in the Introduction, and in concluding chapter, in the American consciousness this is a "redistribution of wealth" and "socialism." The President did not have the guts to assault such a deeply implanted belief.

However the idea of *Medicare For All* is alive. In January 2009, *H.R. 676: The*

---

[*] By the way, it is possible that as a response to Paul Ryan's suggestion that Medicare be partly privatized, many elderly did not vote for Mitt Romney in the 2012 election?

Who Cares about Health Care?

Expanded and Improved Medicare for All Act was introduced in Congress[90] where it has been frozen ever since. People do not know much about it. As a single payer "public option," it is unacceptable to Republicans and desirable but dangerously radical for Democrats.

The summary of the legislation gives enough information for us to understand that this program, as presented, cannot be embraced by Americans.[91]

To begin with, upon enrollment *no* social security number will be required. American citizens and legal aliens do have social security numbers. Is not this an invitation for illegal immigrants?

The new Medicare would cover a host of possible health care issues, including prescription drugs, long-term care, hearing and dental services, drug rehabilitation, and almost everything else. This is good. Also, like today's Medicare for the elderly, one will be able to visit doctors and hospitals of one's choice.

However, like Canada, all the services that are to be covered will be paid for *completely*, with no room for supplemental insurance. Today's our Medicare covers only 80% of health care bills; France's public system pays for about 75% charges. This is quite reasonable and on par with the best world health care systems. Supplemental for-profit insurance, if it is reasonably regulated and does not overcharge, is a healthy way of preventing moral hazard pandemic in systems that pay for all (Medicaid is one of them). But in the new Medicare, there is no room for supplemental insurance whatsoever.

A positive feature of this program is that it would not be controlled by government but rather by a *Medicare for All Trust Fund*, to which the payroll and tax money would be transferred. The Trust would also negotiate the fees and costs with physicians and drug companies. Would not such a "privatization" be a meaningful thing to do as a very first step toward reforming our existing Medicare? Then all the money would be *ours*, and not a dollar would be spent for patching the government's holes. And, quite possibly, it would cost less.

The Act's authors claim that an average American will pay for health care approximately 1.5 times less than under the today's for-profit system. The savings are supposed to originate from "reduced administration, bulk purchasing, and coordination among providers." The sources of financing are as follows:

• Maintain current federal and state funding for existing health care programs
• Establish an employer/employee payroll tax of 4.75% (which would include the present 1.45% Medicare tax)

• Establish a 5% health tax on the top 5% of income earners and a 10% tax on the top 1% of wage earners
• Establish a 0.25% stock and bond transaction tax
• Close corporate tax loopholes
• Repeal the Bush tax cuts for the highest income earners
•Tax unearned income: gambling, capital gains, or lotteries

To me, as a layman, it is impossible to ascertain whether this suggested financing is realistic. I would like to hear what CBO or RAND would say. Because there has been no discussion of the plan, it is impossible to say how well or badly it would work.

This plan is definitely more radical than Obamacare, and I would say, unnecessary radical. In a democratic state, both plans would have to be presented together and allowed to compete. Which one is better? As a layman, I think that, as Soviet dictator Josef Stalin said in a different context, "Both are worse!"

In my view, a *Medicare for All* system would be more humane and would solve a host of problems Obamacare has been trapped in. But it is not going to happen (at least not now).

In this chapter I shared with my readers how I, as a layman, see our health care system today. Unfortunately, many issues are outside my attention and knowledge. Perhaps, after having traveled with me throughout a few different countries, some readers will agree with what I believe is right. In the next, concluding chapter, I will be discussing the question that I posed in the sub-title of this book: *How Are We Different?*

5. CONCLUSION:

How Are We Different?

> We boil at different degrees.
> *Ralph Waldo Emerson*

In this chapter I will attempt to compare our health care with those of the other six countries we have visited. Our health care has many attractive features and in some aspects it is better than that in the other countries. And yet, let us explore what is worth thinking about in those other countries. In other words, which health care system seems to be the most attractive?

How do I, a layman, understand the "attractiveness" of health care systems in this and other countries? From the moral point of view, a good health care system's first goal must be to help the sick, no matter what. From the economic point of view, the system has to be affordable and stable enough so as not to endanger the economic stability of the nation. From the medical point of view, it has to be efficient enough to meet the needs of the citizenry.

In order to compare some important features of health care systems of other countries, I compiled a table of health care indicators based mostly on OECD data. I referred to it (as "the table") in previous chapters, and now you can find it below.

In a humane society it is natural to begin with

The Moral Factor

A good health care has to be a *right* that the citizens can exercise as naturally as they exercise free speech. Of the six countries we have visited, America is the only country where one's health care is a *commodity*, and an expensive one. Hence tens of millions are uninsured. Obamacare attempted to make this commodity more affordable (at least for some) with its main objective to make health care accessible for all. Although the goal "No Uninsured Left Behind" will not be fully achieved, the reform was a leap towards equitability. With all the controversies and drawbacks of Obamacare, it would be unfair to accuse our post-Obama health care system of being less humane than the health care systems we have visited.

Let me now turn to

Health Care Economics

We spend a good chunk of our GDP on health care: 17.7% – significantly more than the other countries (9.3% on average in OECD countries). However, because we are more affluent, we naturally spend more, as I discussed in the previous chapter: not only on health care but also on everything, simply because our disposable income is higher. In the previous chapter I introduced the *Affluence Factor*, the ratio of U.S. GDP per capita to those of other countries. Adjusting each country's expenses to its AF we can compare "apples to apples." Then, as we can see from the table, the disparity becomes less dramatic between what we spend on health care per capita, out of pocket, on drugs, etc., and what the other countries would spend were they as affluent as we are. Clearly, it would be much less if we got rid of the enormous waste that I discussed in the previous chapter.

However, this trick of mine does not exonerate us from "overspending." In the previous chapter I attempted to analyse possible sources of "money rotting," and was unable to find any major cause, although I did find a huge (close to 30%) waste spread across the board.

In the table below is an important entry: Public spending per capita. "Public" means that the source of payments is the government's budget. We see that in simple dollars, our spending (all kinds of government programs and subsidies) is higher than in other countries. Does it mean that we are "more socialistic" than the others? However, if we do AF corrections (i.e., assume that other countries are as affluent as we are), we will see that we are on par with the others. The entries in the table all were collected before Obamacare. Even then we did not mind paying for significant subsidies. Affordability of health care is a tricky question. In America it is not simple. A large group of people – Medicaid and CHIP beneficiaries, 54 million in 2012, which may swell by 20 million by 2016 to comprise close to 25% of our population,[1,2] – did not and will not pay virtually anything for their health care.

As I discussed in the Obamacare chapter, before ACA, the moment one's income exceeded the Medicaid threshold, even by $1, one fell into a "hole." Being ineligible for government entitlements, millions of people were unable to pay at all and therefore did not have health insurance. Obamacare has changed the situation significantly. Even if an individual or family becomes ineligible

Health Care Indicators[1]

	U.S.A.	Canada	France	Germany	Japan	England	Israel
Total GDP, US $/ capita[2]	51,689	41,455	36,249	41,231	35,207	37,447	29,830
Affluence Factors[3]	1.	1.25	1.43	1.25	1.47	1.38	1.73
Health Expenditure:							
% GDP	17.7	11.2	11.6	11.3	9.6	9.4	7.7
Per capita.total, $/"true $"[4]	8,508/8,508	4,666/5,833	4,118/5,889	4,495/5,619	3,213/4,723	3,405/4,699	2,239/3,873
Per capita public, $/"true $"	4,066/4,066	3,182/3,978	3,160/4,519	3,436/5154	2,638/3,878	2,821/3,893	1,362/2,356
Per capita. Out-of-pocket, $/"true $"	987.4/987.4	699.6/874.5	307.0/439.0	593.4/741.8	463.7/681.6	338.3/466.9	581.6/1,006.2
Drug Expenditure per capita, U.S.$	995.0/995.0[5]	751.5/939.4	641.1/916.8	632.6/790.8	651.6/967.9	374.6/516.9	$316.0[6]/547.0
Physicians/1000 population	2.5	2.4[7]	3.3[7]	3.8	2.2	2.8	3.3
GP/Specialists/Others,%	12.3/65./22.7	47.4/51./1.6	49./46.9/4.1.	18./56.9/25..		29.8/66.1/4.1	20.3/62.1./18.
Nurses//1000 population	11.1	9.3	8.7	11.4	10.0	8.6	4.8
Dentists/100 000 population	60	58	67	77	74	42	107[8]
Physicians visits / capita	4.1	7.4	6.8	9.7	13.1	5.0	6.2
Dentists visits/capita	1.0		1.7	1.4	3.2	0.7	2.3
Number of visits/doctor	1,601	3,164	2,051	2,255	6,129	1,848	1,799
Hospital beds/1000 population	3.1	2.8	6.4	8.3	13.4	3.0	3.3
Average stay in hospital, days	4.9	7.7	5.7	9.5	18.2	7.4	5.8
Psychiatric Care Beds/1000 popul.	0.3	0.4	0.9	1.2	2.7	0.5	0.5
Psychiatrists/1000 population[9]	14.1	15.8	22.1	20.9	11.1	19.5	16.7
Suicide rate/100,000 population[5]	12.5	11.1	16.2	10.8	20.9	6.7	7.4
Life expectancy Female/Male:							
At birth	81.1/76.3	83.3/78.7	85.7/78.7	83.2/78.4	85.9/79.4	83.1/79.1	83.6/79.9
At age 65	20.4/17.8	21.6/18.5	23.8/19.3	21.2/18.2	23.7/18.7	21.2/18.6	21.2/19.0
Infant mortality/1000 live births	6.1	4.9	3.5	3.6	2.3	4.3	3.5
Low birth weight infants, %[10]	8.2	6.0	6.6	7.4	9.6	7.4	8.2
Vaccination % children age 2 pertussis/measles/hepatitis B	83.9/90./92.4	?/?/17.0[11]	99./90./47.[11]	96.8/95.9/90.5	96./93.6/?	95./87./?	95./97./99.
Daily smokers, % of population	14.8	15.7	23.3	21.9	20.1	19.6	18.5
Alcohol consumption, aged 15+ liters	8.6	8.0	12.6	11.7	7.3	10.0	2.4
Female/male:							
Overweight adults, %:[12]	28.2/38.6	30.8/40.9	23.3/37.6	29.1/44.4	27.6/26.8	31.7/41.6	28.0/40.7
Obesity adults,%[6]	36.3/35.5	23.3/25.2	13.4/12.4	13.8/15.7	9.6/3.8	26.1/26.2	14.9/17.1
Obes. children. age 5-17,%[13]	35.9/35.0	26.1/28.9	14.9/13.1	17.6/22.6	14.4/16.2	26.6/22.7	17[14]
Diabetes ages 20-79, %[15]	10.3 (2010)	9.2	5.6	5.5	5.0	5.4	6.5
Children aged 0-14/100,000[16]	23.7		12.2	18.0	2.4	24.5	10.4

Mortality rate/100,000, fems/mls[17]							
Heart attack	68/129	61/123	19/50	56/110	17/38	50/110	43/78
Stroke	29/32	29/34	22/31	32/39	30/53	39/42	23/28
All cancers	130/185	143/205	111/221	121/193	93/189	121/194.0/	125/162
Total transport mortality/homicide[18]	14.6/5.0	8.8/1.8	6.8/1.4	5.0/0.8	4.1/0.5	4.0/1.2	5.9/2.1
Coronary angioplasty/100,000	377	105	194	582		178	198
Five-year breast cancer survival, %[19]	89.3	87.7	82.8	83.3	87.3	80.7	86.1
Cesarean section/100 live births	32.3	26.6	20.0	30.3		23.7	18.8
Hip/knee replacement/100,000	184/213	123/143	224/119	296/213	no data	194/141	51/47
Dementia prevalence among 60 and older, %[5]	6.2	5.7	6.5	5.8	6.1	6.1	5.5
MRI/CT units/million	31.6/40.0	8.2/15.0	7.0/12.5	10.3/17.7	43.1/97.3	5.9/8.2	2.0/9.2
MRI/CT exams/1000	97.7/285.0	43.0/125.4	55.2/138.7	no data	no data	40.8/76.6	18.1/127.2
MRI imaging fee, $/"true $"[42]	1,121/1,121[20]	824/981	363/497[3]	839/1,024	250[21]/353	179/242	No data

[1] Unless given other references, the data are from *OECD Health Data 2013) – Frequently Requested Data.* ("2011 or nearest years." Last updated: January, 2014) http://www.oecd.org/health/health-systems/oecdhealthdata2012-frequentlyrequesteddata.htm

[2] *OECD Stat Extracts, 2012:* http://stats.oecd.org/index.aspx?DataSetCode=DECOMP

[3] Ratio of GDP/capita of the U.S. to that of other countries

[4] Multiplied by Affluence Factors

[5] Approximately 30% of pharmaceutical expenses in the U.S. are covered out of pocket (footnote *)

[6] *OECD Health at a Glance. 2011:* http://apps.who.int/medicinedocs/documents/s19848en/s19848en.pdf

[7] "Data include not only doctors providing direct health care, but also health managers, educators, researchers, etc (adding another 5-10% of doctors)

[8] *Number of Dentists in Israel Decreases:* http://www.dentistrytoday.com/todays-dental-news/6617-number-of-dentists-in-israel-decreases

[9] *Health at a Glance 2013, OECD Indicators:* http://www.oecd-ilibrary.org/social-issues-migration-health/health-at-a-glance 19991312; http://www.oecd.org/els/health-systems/Health-at-a-Glance-2013-Chart-set.pdf

[9] Percent of newborn weighing less than 2,500 g. (5.5lb)

[10] Percent of newborn weighing less than 2,500 g. (5.5lb)

[11] "Not required and not routinely provided at age 2"

[12] *OECD Factbook 2013:* http://www.oecd-ilibrary.org/sites/factbook-2013-en/12/02/03/index.html?itemId=/content/chapter/factbook-2013-100-en

[13] *OECD Obesity Update 2012:* http://www.oecd.org/health/49716427.pdf

[14] Romy Zipkin (July 26, 2013). *Israeli Childhood Obesity Nears American Rates:* http://www.tabletmag.com/scroll/139170/israeli-childhood-obesity-nears-american-rates

[15] *OECD Health at a Glance, Europe 2012:* http://www.oecd.org/health/health-systems/HealthAtAGlanceEurope2012.pdf

[16] First line: diabetes Type 2; second line: Type 1. Both the adults and children data are estimates, 2010

[17] *Health at a Glance. 2011 OECD Indicators:* http://www.oecd.org/health/health-systems/49105858.pdf

[18] *UNODC Homicide Statistics:* http://www.unodc.org/unodc/en/data-and-analysis/homicide.html

[19] *OECD Library. Health at a Glance, 2013:* http://www.oecd-ilibrary.org/social-issues-migration-health/health-at-a-glance-2013/screening-survival-and-mortality-for-breast-cancer_health_glance-2013-52-en; jsessionid=wrtxb3ylrcvx.x-oecd-live-01-cancer_health_glance-2013-52-en;jsessionid=wrtxb3ylrcvx.x-oecd-live-01

[20] *International Federation of Health Plans, 2012 Comparative Price Report:* http://www.ifhp.com/documents/2012iFHPPriceReportFINALMarch25.pdf

[21] Source unreliable

for Medicaid with an income over 138%FPL, tax rebates for those with income up to 400%FPL, and out-of-pocket expense subsidies up to 250%FLP become available. The hole still exists, but it is quite shallow and quickly disappears, smoothly switching to the expenses that higher income people will pay, which are significant. Thus, although ACA made our health care system extremely expensive to run, the health system is now more equitable in that some 30 million more people are eligible for decent health care.

In the American consciousness, taxes are the worst evil possible. We are different from the other countries in that they have *a lot* for their taxes as a source of payment for their health, whereas most Americans pay for their health insurance separately, and pay a significant percentage of their income after taxes: Obamacare's Gold and Platinum plans might cost more than 12.5% of an individual or family budget.[1] We do not consider these expenses as a "tax." Tax or no tax, we pay, and it is obvious that we pay for health care (from the government's or our own pockets) more than do people in other countries.

Thus, from the economic point of view our health care system seems less efficient than others. AF or no AF, other systems spend less. The most economical are Israel, Japan and England.

Let us see how the health care systems compare

Providing Good Care

In discussing this issue I will be moving down the entries of the table. Let us begin with the entry "physicians/1000 population."

We have a shortage of physicians compared with the other countries except for Canada and Japan: 2.5 per 1000 population, and the ratio of specialty doctors to general practitioners is disproportionately high, probably because specialists make more money: some 2. to 2.5 times more depending on the specialty.

Our doctors earn some 5.5 times more than average salaries in America, which is relatively more than other countries pay their doctors. I have discussed that in the previous chapter. Here I only repeat that, even disregarding other factors, we have to pay doctors more because the market dictates it: the supply of physicians does not satisfy the demand.

The shortage of specialty doctors translates into long wait times to see them.

In many OECD countries, it is normal to wait six weeks for heart surgery, and as long as five months for knee or hip replacement. This is typical of the countries where health care is controlled by the government, at least through taxes; among them Canada and the U.K. A few numbers below will show where we are vis-à-vis the delay problems: [2,3]

Percent of patients waiting (2010)	U.S.	Canada	France	Germany	U.K.
Six or more days to see a primary care doctor	19%	32%	17%	16%	8%
Four or more weeks to see a specialist	20%	59%	47%	17%	28%
Four or more months for elective surgery	7%	25%	7%	5% (2007)	21%

We see that in the first and third wait categories we are on par with France and Germany. We have fewer internists: 0.3/1000 population vs. 1.6 in France, and 0.6 in Germany (in the table those numbers are expressed in percents). Hence our waiting for a visit to a PCP is a bit longer, though not proportionally longer. No wonder we wait for a specialist visit less than all the countries except Germany: 65% of our physicians are specialists. In the U.K. there are a bit more specialists: 66%, although the waiting time for an appointment is longer.

On the other hand, our doctors try to avoid specialties that are high risk for malpractice suits. One of the most dangerous is the ob-gyn specialty. As a result, in rural or inner-city neighborhoods pre-natal and post-natal care is poor. Besides, many of the patients are uninsured and the doctors are underpaid. No wonder old doctors speedily retire, and young ones decide to become dermatologists, dentists or other "safer" medical specialists. The other countries we have examined do not have this fear of malpractice.

A feature that is almost completely absent from our health care, but that exists in France, Germany, Israel, Japan, and some provinces in Canada, is doctor's house call. This is an important issue. House calls are not possible in the U.S. because we are extremely short of general practitioners. People with flu and colds come to a doctor's office sneezing and coughing, infecting other patients in waiting room. To say nothing of the fact that driving while sick (especially when people come to see a doctor when they cannot wait any longer) may be dangerous. Unfortunately, nowhere have I found information on what the dollar cost of neglecting that important doctor's function can be; it may be large. It is hoped that the situation may soon change. ACA has a provision called the *Independence at Home Act*. Before it goes into effect, a three-year demonstration project was initiated in 2012. "Under this Demonstration, 10,000 home-limited Medicare beneficiaries with multiple chronic conditions will be provided longitudinal primary care and care coordination services by teams of physician or nurse practitioner-headed provider groups."[4]

In France and Germany doctors often make house calls outside normal working hours, even at night. At that time of day Americans call emergency. Fortunately, our 911 services are good, although one often has to wait a long time once having arrived at an emergency room.[*] One of the reasons for the wait is that people without health insurance often rush to emergency rooms with issues that either could have been easily resolved by a PCP, to whom they do not have access, or already serious enough to require hospitalization. Our emergency service is, however, fundamentally different from that in France and Germany where in life-threatening cases a doctor, rather than a paramedic, comes to the patient, and, if possible, begins treatment before the patient is moved to an emergency room or a hospital.[†]

We have more nurses per 1000 population than all countries except England. As I mentioned in the previous chapter, nurses often do physicians' work, which partly compensates for the shortage of physicians, although sometimes it may be counter-productive. Unfortunately, both in the U.S. and other countries, because of the current economic crises, the remuneration of nurses has been cut down. This problem has not affected physicians.

Only Canada and England have fewer dentists than we have. However, to have an appointment with a dentist is not a problem in most cases. And here I want to mention a serious drawback of the American health care system, which I discussed in the previous chapter. In all the countries we have visited (except Canada) dental care is covered either completely or in large part. In America one has to purchase separate and expensive dental insurance that insufficiently covers dental work. Until recently, coverage for implants has been out of the question. Only 50% of people of low income (but not low enough to be eligible for Medicaid) visit a dentist unless their toothache is unbearable. Medicaid, however, completely pays for any dental work. Orthodontic care for children and teenagers is mostly paid from their parents' pockets. How Obamacare will resolve this long neglected problem is still in fog.

Americans visit doctors' offices less frequently than do patients in other

---

[*] Hence a "commandment": If the issue is serious, do not take the patient to an ER; call 911: then the ambulance will bring the patient directly to the appropriate hospital department, avoiding spending a long time in an ER.
[†] Remember Princess Diana's accident controversy?

countries. This is probably because almost any visit to a doctor requires a co-payment, and a large bill will follows a dentist's visit. In other countries people do not think twice before going to a doctor, and this is a consequence of moral hazard: "Why not visit a doctor if everything will be paid for no matter what?"

We have fewer hospital beds per 1000 population than the other countries, especially France, Germany and Japan. Yet, our hospitals are less crowded: a semi-private room for two is typical. Also, at least in the Greater Boston area where I live, I have not heard of cases when people had to wait to be accepted to a hospital. However, Boston is one of the medical capitals of the world. In other areas the situation may be different. Staying in a hospital in America, however, is extremely and unexplainably expensive, which adds-up to our health care cost. Japan has over four times more hospital beds than the U.S., and patients stay there some three times longer than here. The elderly in Japan prefer staying in hospitals rather than moving to nursing homes.

Our hospital stays are shorter than in Canada, Germany, Japan, and England, not only because they are astronomically expensive and because insurance companies restrict the number of days they pay for. American medical strategy dictates that patients begin recovery after surgery as quickly as possible – at home. This is good. It also helps to avoid nasty infections often contracted in hospitals. Poor hospital hygiene in American hospitals still remains a significant problem. Doctors sometimes fail to disinfect their stethoscopes, which can be the source of serious infections.[*]

The next entry is about the current state of psychiatric care. In the previous chapter I discussed our failure to take care of mental illnesses. We are failing to deliver high-quality psychiatric care because of our irresponsible attitude towards psychiatric disorders; they are either not covered by insurance policies or covered incompletely. Among the countries we have visited, only Canada does not pay for treatment of mental illnesses from its Medicare coffers. France covers 70% of treatment costs from the "public option," but inexpensive supplemental insurance picks up the bills. We have fewer psychiatric care beds in our hospitals and fewer psychiatrists than the other countries discussed. Japan is an abnormality: it has a greater number of psychiatric beds, fewer psychiatrists, and an enormous suicide rate: almost twice that of the U.S. and the other countries, apart from Israel. In Israel the suicide rate is half that of the U.S. An Israeli anomaly: "A new study shows them to be among the most contented in the Western world,"[5]And that is in spite of enormous stress of living under the thread of annihilation!

A black spot on the reputation of America's health care is our lower life

---

[*] The excellent book by Dr. Atul Gawande, *Complication*, discusses this issue.

expectancy and higher infant mortality than in other OECD countries. Let us begin with life expectancy.

In January 2013, when this book was almost finished, a report (*U.S. Health in International Perspective: Shorter Lives, Poorer Health*) was issued by the National Institutes of Health.[6] The report provoked a nation-wide response by the media. The main causes of our low life expectancy and poor health were identified as infant mortality and low birth weight, injuries and homicides, adolescent pregnancy and sexually transmitted infections, HIV and AIDS, drug-related deaths, obesity[*] and diabetes, heart disease, chronic lung disease and disability. In this chapter I discuss most of these factors. Both the report and this book used the same data from 2012 OECD Health care Indicators.[†1]

In my view, our health care system is not completely responsible for Americans' lower life expectancy. As we saw when discussing Canada, a significant percentage of the mortality gap for adults in their twenties can be explained by the higher American accident/homicide rates. Living in America, one "is four times more likely to be murdered than if one lives in Britain, almost six times more likely than in Germany, and 13 times more likely than in Japan." The table shows these impressive statistics.

For people over 50, the difference in mortality rates is due to the larger number of people with cardiovascular disease in the U.S., which is more likely a result of unhealthy lifestyle rather than inefficiency of the health care system. Obamacare will provide a range of preventive measures, which would affect the incidence of all illnesses, including cardio-vascular diseases.

It is also interesting to compare the life expectancy of people at the age of 65 who have already survived crazy drivers and stray bullets. From the table we see that American elderly live almost as long as their peers in the other countries. Is it because Medicare takes care of them well?

Actually, it is not quite right to compare the U.S. to homogeneous populations of other countries because we have a mixture of ethnic groups and cultures. However, ethnicity and social factors alone cannot explain the higher mortality rate in America. When millions of people have poor access to good health

---

[*] Quite unexpectedly, as published in the January 2013 issue of Journal of American Medical Association, a detailed analysis of combined data of 97 studies throughout the world found that very mild, "grade1," obesity (body-mass index, BMI between 30 and 35 kg/m^2) "was not associated with increased all-cause mortality". (Lesser degrees of excess weight don't increase mortality http://www.medscape.com/viewarticle/791407).

[†] I have made the necessary updates to the data when 2013 OECD Health Care Indicators became available.

care, it is quite likely that they would not be living long.

In the previous chapter I discussed some factors responsible for high infant mortality such as our poor maternity and vaccination regulations. However, to blame our health care alone for high infant mortality does not seem right.

I discussed this issue in detail when I was comparing Canada with the U.S. Let us look at the *Low birth weight infant* data in the table. Together with Israel, we have the highest percentage of newborn babies weighing less than 5.5 lbs. (Japan is the first; but the Japanese are, on average, smaller people and that could be an explanation.) American doctors fight for the lives of babies no matter how small, premature, or even born with birth defects. Those efforts are unequalled elsewhere. That is why there are more such babies born in the U.S. than in the other countries we visited and in about 30 OECD developed countries.[1] However, in spite of the selfless efforts of our doctors, low birth weight babies die more frequently than normal birth weight babies. This has nothing to do with the health care system. Also, the methodology of counting premature babies varies in different countries. Only eight countries (including the U.S.) count premature babies that have a low chance for survival as live births[7]; hence the statistics placing America close to Belarus.

As for Israel, in spite of the high percentage of low birth weight infants, its infant mortality is almost twice as low as ours. This is a manifestation of superb neonatal care in Israel.

As I discussed in the previous chapter, vaccination regulations in the U.S. are insufficient, which has already resulted in a resurgence of illnesses we believed to have been eradicated.

Now let us see how our system compares in approaching the most serious health issues.

Smoking is gradually disappearing from America's social life. Unfortunately, popularity of e-cigarettes, especially among children, grows:

> ...the US Centers for Disease Control and Prevention reported that the percentage of middle and high school students who used had more than doubled between 2011 and 2012 in the USA, and one in five middle school children who reported using e-cigarettes had never smoked conventional cigarettes.[*8]

Also, a 2011 Center for Disease Control's studies have found that young

---

[*] According to the 2013 US National Youth Tobacco Survey, using e-cigarettes by young people increased dramatically from 79 000 in 2011, to 263 000 in 2013 (http://ntr.oxfordjournals.org/content/early/2014/08/18/ntr.ntu166).

women smoke a lot: 1 in 6 women, age 18 and older, smoke cigarettes.[9] This has nothing to do with any drawbacks of our health care system per se, although it will have serious consequences if we are in fact facing a smoke-related cancer epidemic among women, as the above source claims. Fortunately, keen health care awareness is a part of our culture. The threat of lung cancer has caused millions of people to quit smoking.[*]

America consumes less alcohol than the other countries (but not Israel, which is a champion of sobriety!). We mostly drink beer. Germany and England also drink beer, and they are champions of beer drinking.[†] The French prefer wine and drink a lot of it! This is believed to be a major factor in their reduced incidence of heart disease.

Now, a gloomy indicator. In the previous chapter I referenced the Commonwealth Fund spending analysis,[10] which mentioned obesity as one of the three most important factors of America's "overspending." We have an epidemic of overweight and obesity, which has obvious causes: unhealthy lifestyle and unhealthy food. We spend hours in front of the TV, or surfing the Web, or playing video and computer games. The food industry, matching our life-style, supplies us in abundance with fast food, which is not always healthy.

The most dramatic, if not tragic, aspect of this epidemic is that it is spreading to children. Look at the table: our children are the fattest among their peers in other countries! They do not play outside with their friends as they used to do decades ago. They sit at their play stations or computers for hours. It is commonly believed that computers are good for intellectual development. However, there are reliable data that indicate that computers are not as good for children's education as believed, but I do not intend to discuss this at length.[‡]

In Japan, mandatory obesity screening is administered. We do not do this.

---

[*] It took decades to force tobacco companies to acknowledge that they had been concealing the connection of lung cancer with smoking. As I mentioned discussing health care in Nazi Germany, the Nazis were the first to establish that connection. However, after Germany's collapse in 1945, the victors, presumably in order to preserve the enormous profits of tobacco companies, deliberately hid that information.

[†] A German friend has told me that on Friday nights in Munich, where he lives, the police are overwhelmed by phone calls reporting stolen cars. Of course, after having drunk a gallon of beer not many can remember where they parked their cars!

[‡] Just a short note: We confuse information with knowledge. Computers allow easy access to information; however, transforming information into knowledge requires serious and time-consuming intellectual work. Unfortunately, our kids are not encouraged to work hard: computers make everything easy. Some Silicone Valley parents are against it; see "A Valley School That Doesn't Compute:" http://www.lemproject.eu/in-focus/news/a-silicon-valley-school-that-doesn2019t-compute.

Conclusion: How Are We Different?

Should our health care system be excused for not preventing people from adding pounds? Disease prevention is a part of medicine. Health clinics exist that have diabetes rooms to give individual advice regarding diet, exercise, even preventative treatment for people with a genetically identified risk. And yet these efforts are not enough to stop the obesity epidemic. Doctors do encourage healthy lifestyle and good nutrition (or a radical surgery in special cases). However they may not recommend a diet as a part of treatment; partly because few American doctors are educated in nutrition, and some dismiss it as a new-age nonsense.

Diets have been overtaken by the media and commercialized. Unfortunately, not enough research is being done to ascertain which diets are good and which are bad or useless. Generally, Americans are receptive to advice and are compliant; we witness the significant reduction in smoking, the popularity of fitness centers, or adjusting food pyramid without any diets. However, as in the case of smoking, overweight and obesity are generally outside the health care system. I do not think we can administer obesity screening, as it is done in Japan. In the U.S. this may be considered a violation of an individual liberty (to be fat!).

Diabetes follows obesity, and here we are also champions.[*] However, the awareness of the danger of both obesity and diabetes is growing in America, and the ACA should take this issue seriously.

The table's next two entries are the number one killers: cardiovascular diseases (heart attacks and strokes). Here we are again ahead of the others. There are quite a few factors that contribute to cardiovascular diseases, among them overweight, unhealthy diet, stress, and other social issues. Awareness of symptoms enables early intervention. Interventional cardiology that mends clogged arteries has saved thousands of lives. The U.S. is a pioneer in such procedures. A patient with suspicious heart attack symptoms can be transferred to an operating room right from an ambulance. Most hospitals have cardiovascular teams. The number of coronary angioplasty procedures (placing stents into clogged arteries – an efficient substitute for coronary bypass) in America is higher than in the other countries, apart from Germany (and there it is gigantic!).

France performs only half the number of angioplasty procedures that we do. Why? Look at the number of heart attacks that the French suffer: it is 3.5 times less for women and 2.5 times less for men than among Americans. They do

---

[*] This is Type 2 diabetes that follows obesity. Type 1 diabetes is a genetic autoimmune illness. It usually begins in childhood or adolescence: the immune system begins destroying the pancreatic cells that create insulin.

205

not need angioplasties: their hearts are healthier! Is it partly because they drink a lot of wine? Or because the life in a welfare state is less stressful?

In America, the symptoms of stroke are now known nationally. An acronym, F.A.S.T.[*][11] helps victims and observers memorize the stroke symptoms and act immediately. On TV news and on the Web, people are advised to have an aspirin ready to take immediately when the symptoms appear. Bayer aggressively advertises aspirinas as the first aid. This advice, however is wrong.

The thing is that "there are two kinds of strokes: ischemic stroke, caused by a clot that blocks a blood vessel supplying the brain with blood, and hemorrhagic or bleeding stroke, caused by a leaky blood vessel that bleeds into the brain." [12] If a stroke is hemorrhagic then thinning the blood by taking aspirin worsens the situation, and may result in death. Conversely, in the case of an ischemic event where a blood vessel is clotted the use of drugs to thin the blood is appropriate and often necessary. Only a doctor can diagnose stroke correctly. A CT scan of the head can help determine if a stroke is ischemic or hemorrhagic. Timing is critical in relation to outcomes, therefore at the first signs of stroke immediately call 911. Even in small towns, paramedics arrive within a very short time when a heart attack or stroke is suspected.

The 2000 World Health Organization's health-care ranking assigned the U.S. No.37 among 190 nations. France was No.1. As I discuss in the introduction to Chapter 2, the most recent (2013) Bloomberg rankings: *The World's Most Efficient Health Care Systems*, and *The World's Healthiest Countries*[13] pushed France respectively to No.19 and No.13, while the U.S. were No. 46 and No. 33. I could not find detailed data of how those places had been awarded. However, I would like to note, that what brought us down in the WHO's ranking: No.54-55 was in the category *Fairness In Financial Contributions*. In *Health Level* we were No.24, a bit lower than Germany (No.22). However, the category *Responsiveness Level* awards us No.1, while France was No.3.[14]

These numbers show that when it comes to diagnosing and treating illnesses the U.S. is not at the bottom of the list. As an example: we are first in five-year breast cancer survival. Cancer awareness is very high in the American consciousness today.

---

[*] "*Face:* Ask the person to smile. Does one part of the face droop? *Arms:* Ask the person to raise both arms. Does one arm drifts downward? *Speech:* Ask the person to repeat a simple phrase. Is the speech slurred or strange? *Time:* If you observe one of these signs call 911 immediately. One in three Americans can identify any of the symptoms."

Conclusion: How Are We Different?

The next entry is the number of cesarean sections performed. Here we are the champion (with Germany at our heels). This is a multi-faceted issue; I discussed it in detail in the previous chapter.

In the table I also included an indicator of interest to me as well as to millions of people in the same – elderly – club: the numbers of hip and knee replacements per 100,000 population. As one can see, we are on par with almost all the other countries. For some reason, Israel is well behind. This is another Israeli "abnormality" that is not easy to explain.

In the previous chapter I discussed in detail Alzheimer's disease, the illness I believe is threatening the very existence of our civilization. The table contains the data on the prevalence of dementia among those aged 60 and older. We are, more or less, on par with the other countries. Israel has the lowest dementia incidence.

Long-term care is probably the most acute problem of health care because the elderly are about to "invade" the world, bringing with them Alzheimer's and other debilitating illnesses. In the countries we have visited, LTC is provided in various ways. However, home care over facility-based care is the main principle around which all the rather complex LTC systems revolve. I discussed our LTC in the previous chapter. Unfortunately, in this area we are behind the other countries.

Next in the table are two indicators that have to do with the most advanced diagnostic techniques: MRI/CT. In numbers of operational MRI/CT units we are behind only Japan. Canada has three times fewer MRI/CT machines per million population than the U.S. However, although those numbers are larger than in France (8.2/15.0 vs. 7.0/12.5), the machines are used less efficiently: 43.0/125.5 exams per 1000 population vs. 55.2/138.7 exams in France. The imaging fee in France is almost twice as low as that in Canada. Our MRI imaging fee is higher than in the other countries, even if their fees are corrected for AF. This is because all our MRI machines belong to for-profit clinics; these clinics also purchase machines from manufacturers for higher prices than in Europe. All the high-tech equipment and new drugs are more expensive in the U.S. than in other countries. Most probably it is because prices in other countries are strongly regulated by the governments; therefore companies manufacturing advanced equipment and drugs try to get the desired profit in the U.S. with no government interference. As a result, the costs reflecting the double profit trickle down to our bills.

The table is over.

Here I would like to say a few words about a leading American national laboratory, the National Institutes of Health (NIH), which is an inalienable part of the U.S. health care system. * While it takes in $35 billion from the government budget, at the same time it provides new ideas and technological innovations in health care. It is difficult to overestimate the impact that NIH has not only on America's health care but also on the economy in general. National Institute of Health has a huge portfolio of patents and licenses instrumental in the development of new medical technologies and drugs. Especially important is NIH's role in developing and promoting therapeutics for treating cancers and developing vaccines for preventing infectious diseases. The transfer of technology from NIH both to American private businesses and to other countries through broad international collaboration also cannot be underestimated. In April, 2013, NIH launched a ten year BRAIN (Brain Research through Advancing Innovative Neurotechnologies) Initiative "to revolutionize the understanding of the human brain,"[15] which is expected to make a significant contribution to understanding Alzheimer's disease.

I hope that I have provided some food for thought while discussing the above "attractiveness criteria." Let me now discuss the one million dollar question:

Which Health Care Seems Most Attractive?

In my view it is the French one, even if it was "de-crowned" by the Bloomberg. Of course, the French system cannot be copied in America. The French economy and its health care are in deep financial crisis, and in the near future the system will have to undergo a great deal of change, probably for the worse. However, the French have developed a system that should be studied if we seriously want to understand how our own system can be improved.

Researching the Web, I have found claims that the French and the American health care systems have much in common: "twins separated at birth."[16] Let me repeat the quote with which I finished the chapter on France:

> Several salient features of the French health care system – the dominance of office-based private practice (la médecine libérale) for ambulatory care, the mix of public and private hospitals, the widespread use of cost sharing, the predominant practice of direct payment from patient to doctor, and the reliance upon financing derived from payroll taxes – resemble elements of the U.S. health system. These points of convergence make French national health insurance especially relevant to Americans interested in learning from abroad.[17]

---

* I am grateful to my friend Lev Goldfarb, M.D., for bringing my attention to the impact of NIH on our health care and economy.

However, the French health care system is much less expensive. Below is the table that shows a few indicators of its cost (the first two are also in the table on pp. 218-219):[18] The last column shows how much we would pay were we less affluent, as France is. Not much relief! We would spend less only from government's pocket.

	FRANCE ($)	USA ($)	USA Devided by AF=1.43
Spending/costs:			
Total health spending/capita[xiv]	3,160.	8,508.	5,950.
Public (govt) spending/capita	3,269.	4,066.	2,843.
Doctor's office visit	30.	95.	66.
Stay in hospital/day	853.	4,287.	2,998.
Surgeries (total costs):			
Appendectomy	4,436.	13,851.	9,686.
Child delivery (normal)	3,541.	9,775.	6,822.
Hip replacement	10,927.	40,346.	28,214
C-section	6,441.	15,041.	10,518
Cataract removal	1,938.	3,738.	2,614
Coronary bypass	22,844.	73,420.	51,343.
Angioplasty	7,567.	28,128.	19,670.
Tests:			
CT scan abdominal	183.	630.	441.
CT scan head	183.	566.	396.
Angiogram	264.	914.	639.
MRI	363.	1,121.	784
Cymbolta	47.	176.	123.
Lipitor	48.	124.	87
Nexium	30.	202.	141.
Nasonex	17.	108.	76.

Not only the French system is less expensive; it is also more efficient. If you look at what the French purchase for their money (the list in the France chapter[19]), you will see that virtually all aspects of health care are taken care of, even those that in America are either poorly covered (mental disorders), or need special and expensive insurance (dental and vision).

It is often claimed that the French system is socialistic. The French reject this accusation because their health care, unlike that of England, is virtually independent of government: most of their physicians and many of their hospitals are private. But it is a "single payer" system: no insurance companies are involved, and financial exchanges are realized between patients and their nonprofit health funds.

However, France is a welfare state. Significant resources are spent by the government on health care of the poor. This is the France's "welfareness" that is confused with socialism.

Let us see who the "poor" are in France.[*] Officially, they are those whose income is below the level of poverty (FrPL), which is defined as 50% of median income. There are some 4.9 million of these people (7.5% of the population). In 2012, the FrPL for a single person was $12,348/year (ours was $11,700). Almost free health care covers those below 120%FrPL (60% of median income) i.e., $14,818 (roughly 14% of the population).[†]

Now, what is the situation in the U.S.? According to the 2013 Census Bureau report, in 2011, the official poverty rate (those whose incomes was below the American Federal Poverty Level, AFPL) in the U.S. was 15%:[20] twice that of France. Those people – close to 55 million – are eligible for Medicaid and CHIP, and even before Obamacare, they did receive significant subsidies. In this respect, America was more "welfarish" than France, providing virtually free health care to a higher percentage of the population than in France. Obamacare extends the Medicaid eligibility up to 138%AFPL: for a single, up to $15,414; France's 120%FPL threshold is $14,818 Comparing these numbers we see that, in Obamacare era, we will be spending more per capita on completely subsidized health care than France.

Now when we talk about French "socialism," we should not forget that we are also on par with France when comparing the costs of total subsidies of the poor per capita. France pays government subsidies to 50% of its population. In the Obamacare America people with income below 400% FPL will be receiving either complete (Medicaid) or some government subsidies. To understand how comprehensive those subsidies will be, I used the most recently available (2012) income distribution numbers from the 2011 Census Bureau Survey.[36] Anyone can check these numbers. Even though they are from 2011, they are reliable: In future years the income distribution will most likely be skewed towards lower incomes. The numbers I found are striking. These benefits would be given to 49.0% of the American population. Among two-member families 59% would receive subsistence, and among four-member families it would be 65.5%. These numbers relate only to health care, leaving aside other welfare subsidies.

The expansion of Medicaid and other subsidies will significantly increase

---

[*] I am grateful to my French friend Romuald Ripon for providing me with information available on French language sites. I have also learned to use the GOOGLE translator!

[†] "Almost free" because, as I discussed in the chapter on France, those people do pay, albeit insignificantly, for their health care through taxes and payroll deductions – something that our Medicaid beneficiaries do not do.

government's (i.e., taxpayers') spending. Without such measures the "hole" I discussed above would still exist, and it would be impossible for those low-income people to purchase insurance on market (now called Exchange), because health insurance is still a very expensive commodity. Then, even partly achieving the reform's main goal: "No Uninsured Left Behind" would be impossible.

Unfortunately, expanded welfare has the tendency to reproduce itself because the handouts discourage people from becoming self-sufficient. France is a perfect welfare state. Unless *we, the people*, watch very carefully, America is very likely to copy France in that respect.

So much for the so–called French "socialism."

Let us see what is "good" about France apart from its favorable health care economics. In the table you could see that in many areas France is either better or on par with us. Unlike Americans, who cannot stop criticizing their own health care system (and unfortunately they are right), the French are proud of theirs. Remember, the three symbols of the French nation: "the flag, health and the *Marseillaise*"? It sounds a bit hokey, but that's how they feel.

The main difference between the French system and ours is that, as I have already stressed, the French consider their health care as an inalienable right, albeit heavily paid for. We lack the fundamental ideological notion that the French have: *solidarity*, which, in the context of health care, means that all the people agree voluntarily and without reservation to pay for maintaining the health of everyone else, not only their own. This is imbedded in the consciousness of the nation. Possibly over a half Americans are against such a "re-distribution of wealth;" however as we have seen, we pay for "someone else" more than the French do.

Recently, a distinguished TV journalist whom I respect said that since he had enrolled in Medicare his bills had been paid by his children. In his view, this was a kind of redistribution of wealth, and, as a feature of "socialism," it was bad. But should not children cover a part of their parents' (and grandparents') health care expenses while paying for their own? Should not it be natural that children attempt, however partially and possibly minimally, to pay off the huge debt (both monetary and moral) they owe to those who brought them up?

Another crucial difference is that in France for-profit insurance companies do not "run the show," although they have a for-profit niche providing supplemental insurance. In the previous chapter we saw that for-profit insurers in America do not make that much profit. However, they are bad because the ability to make profit on health care motivates them to minimize expenses, preventing millions of Americans from receiving adequate health care.

Although the ACA somewhat restricted the power of insurance companies to run the show, it has not taken the most important step: forcing insurance companies to forfeit their rights to set rates and to determine cost-sharing amounts (i.e., deductibles, co-payments, and lifetime limits).

Would they agree to that? Competition means that some insurance companies manage to pay for services less than others, or refuse to pay for some services.[*] This is possible either because they do not pay some bills or cut down on their administrative expenses. If they cannot avoid paying all the bills because the standardized tariffs dictate how much *must* be paid (provided, of course, that a more or less universal Health Basket exists) then there will be no difference between non-profits and for-profits, except that the latter will be more expensive to run because they still somehow (by cutting some corners?) would have to make a profit. What I want to say is that if the conditions necessary for achieving universal and fair coverage are imposed on for-profit insurance companies that will be their deathblow. The ACA requires that non-profit and for-profit companies exist together in the same business. I do not understand how this can happen in a state of honest competition.

Concluding...

While attempting to answer the question *How Are We Different?* I could not stop thinking about Richard Nixon's health care reform. America lost the chance of implementing it 40 years ago. Even if the system had bugs, we had plenty of time to fix them. Nixon did not want to destroy for-profit insurance, but he was a humanist who understood the necessity of health-care-for-all. He understood that no economic, racial, or social barriers should stand in the way of good health care. That was the objective of his reform. In 1974, this amounted to a revolution. If the Nixon reform had been implemented, we would be ahead of Europe. Now, in many respects, we are behind.

Two powerful factors: the miserable state of the American economy with our

---

[*] Medscape.com, an authoritative source of Internet information for both doctors and patients, in its entry (http://www.medscape.com/viewarticle/767910?src=mp&spon=38) quotes Dick Browne, Green Cross of Wisconsin's CEO: "a top-to-bottom review of our operations revealed that we were incurring huge costs dealing with angry patients and doctors. Worst of all, giving a reason for denying a claim was simply providing patients with ammunition to argue with us; appeals were hurting our bottom line." Therefore a completely new category of claim denial was announced: *Just Because!* The beauty of *Just Because* according to Browne was that it stopped the appeal process dead in its tracks. And, according to an independent audit, downsizing the appeals could save Green Cross millions.

skyrocketing debt and the skyrocketing cost of high quality health care should have prevented us from doing anything radical. In 1974 Nixon believed that "we should capitalize on the skills and facilities already in place, not replace them and start from scratch with a huge federal bureaucracy to add to the ones we already have." This would be the right strategy today. Unfortunately, we have failed to follow his advice.

In decreasing the number of uninsured, the extension of eligibility for Medicaid will do the main job. Using the Census Bureau population survey[36] I found that some 23 million people will have incomes between 100%AFPL and 138%AFPL and would be eligible for Medicaid (e.g., be given virtually free health insurance) if all the states would agree to expand coverage. (RAND corporation[21] estimates that by 2019 only about 12 million people will join Medicaid; CBO's estimate[15] is 16 million.) Many more people – 81.6 million with incomes between 138%FPL and 400%FPL – will receive some assistance (tax credits and subsidies for out-of-pocket expenses). The system of subsidies and penalties is quite sophisticated – hence an enormous new bureaucracy: See the list of new bureaucratic entities in the Obamacare chapter.

Because of the exorbitant price tags on health insurance, many people were unable to purchase it. I do not want to be misunderstood. Those people must be helped, either through subsidies or by forcing insurance companies – to put their policies on permanent sale. Obamacare chose the first option – hence the enormous expense. This decision, apart from a justifiable humanitarian reason, had a political underpinning: expanding the number of people depending on some form of government handout. As I already mentioned, those with incomes below 400%FLP comprise almost half of our population: 49.0%.

What in my layman's view, could have been accomplished had we followed Richard Nixon's advice?

To begin with, by prohibiting insurance companies from discriminating against pre-existing conditions and other "undesirable" illnesses, some 9 to 12.5 million people (25% to 35% of those who attempted to purchase insurance directly from insurance companies) would be insured.[22,23] Another 2.5 million (young adults up to age 26) would have been insured together with their parents.[24] Thus, even without a new bureaucracy and the creation of a new and complicated system, some 12 - 15 million people might have been insured.

Another option to provide millions of uninsured people with high quality health care is developing a wide network of Community Health Centers. Many people do not even know that these centers exist. In 2013, 22 million Americans depended on these centers' services (some of them were middle class). Patients are charged on a sliding income scale. At the HealthWorks

---

center in Leesburg, Virginia, patients with incomes below 200%AFPL ($47,100 for a family of four), pay for a doctor visit on average $20 to $30. Those with high insurance deductibles pay $60.[25] And, as a Stanford University study showed, the quality of care in such centers are on par with that rendered by private doctors.

Increasing the number of Community Health Centers is within the scope of the ACA. By 2015, over 30 million of Americans would have to be treated there. Originally the ACA allocated $11 billion over five years for these centers. This amount was later slashed to $8 billion; as a result 5 million new patients will not have access to affordable health care. Eight and even $11 billion cannot be compared with the ACA's price tag of close to $500 billion exchange subsidies. According to a CBO report, IRS would have to spend between $5 and $10 billion only to implement ACA![15]

We can see that only expansion of Community Health Centers with no new bureaucracies, regulations, or enormous spending would be a tremendous leap towards a more equitable and efficient health care system.

The rest – including necessary financial assistance to the uninsured – could be accomplished much more effectively through independent state health care programs without federal government interference or control.

As I already mentioned, in 2009, three states: Maine, Massachusetts and Vermont, had already implemented their own reforms that achieved almost universal coverage of their residents. At that time 14 more states were considering comprehensive reforms.[26] Each state would take care of its own finances (with possible government support), and then we would not have to borrow the enormous amount of money that brought us to the edge of the fiscal cliff.

If we had followed this scenario, we would have created a conglomerate of independent state-based health care systems, rather than a federal behemoth forcing states to accept its rules and imposing its control. President Obama could have encouraged and supported such measures but he has not.

Now it is history. ACA is the "Law of the Land," and may remain so (though possibly modified) for years to come. We do not know how it will work and how America will be able to pay its enormous health care bills.

Even if one completely disregards today's idealistic notion that, in a humane society, universal and affordable health care is supposed to be the right of every person, rather than a privilege dependent on one's ability to pay bills, one should not forget that without a form of universal health care our society will eventually have lost its honorable title "humane."

Conclusion: How Are We Different?

No amount of money can prevent death. Death equalizes everybody by a universal action—destruction of the personal universe. Before G-d, all the dying are equal. For the beloved of the dying, it is always an irreparable loss, a tragedy that the brain refuses to comprehend, an event that terminates the previous well-organized life, and an ordeal that may never be overcome. The suffering of the rich is neither worse nor more important than that of the humble poor. That is why nobody has the right to refuse treatment to the sick. Even though this notion may seem to be too radical for our society today, I hope many of my readers will agree with me that it is true. It has definitely something to do with the notion of the responsibility of being one's brother's keeper and the French concept of Solidarity. The need for universal health care will become increasingly pressing with the aging of our society, and we will eventually need to develop a humane and optimal universal health care system.

March 2010 – Dec. 2013.

Peabody, MA

RICHARD NIXON
XXXVII *President of the United States: 1969-1974*

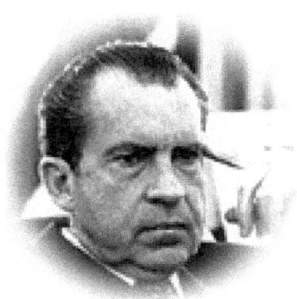

President Nixon's Special Message to the Congress
Proposing a Comprehensive Health Insurance Plan

February 6, 1974

To the Congress of the United States:

One of the most cherished goals of our democracy is to assure every American an equal opportunity to lead a full and productive life.

In the last quarter century, we have made remarkable progress toward that goal, opening the doors to millions of our fellow countrymen who were seeking equal opportunities in education, jobs and voting.

Now it is time that we move forward again in still another critical area: health care.

Without adequate health care, no one can make full use of his or her talents and opportunities. It is thus just as important that economic, racial and social barriers not stand in the way of good health care as it is to eliminate those barriers to a good education and a good job.

Three years ago, I proposed a major health insurance program to the Congress, seeking to guarantee adequate financing of health care on a nationwide basis. That proposal generated widespread discussion and useful debate. But no legislation reached my desk.

Today the need is even more pressing because of the higher costs of medical care. Efforts to control medical costs under the New Economic Policy have been inept with encouraging success, sharply reducing the rate of inflation for health care. Nevertheless, the overall cost of health care has still risen by more than 20 percent in the last two and one-half years, so that more and more Americans face staggering bills when they receive medical help today:

--Across the Nation, the average cost of a day of hospital care now exceeds $110. --The average cost of delivering a baby and providing postnatal care approaches $1,000. --The average cost of health care for terminal cancer now exceeds $20,000.

For the average family, it is clear that without adequate insurance, even normal care can be a financial burden while a catastrophic illness can mean catastrophic debt.

Beyond the question of the prices of health care, our present system of health care insurance suffers from two major flaws:

First, even though more Americans carry health insurance than ever before, the 25 million Americans who remain uninsured often need it the most and are most unlikely to obtain it. They include many who work in seasonal or transient occupations, high-risk cases, and those who are ineligible for Medicaid despite low incomes.

Second, those Americans who do carry health insurance often lack coverage, which is balanced, comprehensive and fully protective:

--Forty percent of those who are insured are not covered for visits to physicians on an out-patient basis, a gap that creates powerful incentives toward high cost care in hospitals;

--Few people have the option of selecting care through prepaid arrangements offered by Health Maintenance Organizations so the system at large does not benefit from the free choice and creative competition this would offer;

--Very few private policies cover preventive services;

--Most health plans do not contain built-in incentives to reduce waste and inefficiency. The extra costs of wasteful practices are passed on, of course, to consumers; and

--Fewer than half of our citizens under 65--and almost none over 65--have major medical coverage which pays for the cost of catastrophic illness.

These gaps in health protection can have tragic consequences. They can cause people to delay seeking medical attention until it is too late. Then a medical crisis ensues, followed by huge medical bills--or worse. Delays in treatment can end in death or lifelong disability.

COMPREHENSIVE HEALTH INSURANCE PLAN (CHIP)

Early last year, I directed the Secretary of Health, Education, and Welfare to prepare a new and improved plan for comprehensive health insurance. That plan, as I indicated in my State of the Union message, has been developed and I am presenting it to the Congress today. I urge its enactment as soon as possible.

The plan is organized around seven principles:

First, it offers every American an opportunity to obtain a balanced, comprehensive range of health insurance benefits;

Second, it will cost no American more than he can afford to pay;

Third, it builds on the strength and diversity of our existing public and private systems of health financing and harmonizes them into an overall system;

Fourth, it uses public funds only where needed and requires no new Federal taxes;

Fifth, it would maintain freedom of choice by patients and ensure that doctors work for their patient, not for the Federal Government.

Sixth, it encourages more effective use of our health care resources;

And finally, it is organized so that all parties would have a direct stake in making the system work--consumer, provider, insurer, State governments and the Federal Government.

BROAD AND BALANCED PROTECTION FOR ALL AMERICANS

Upon adoption of appropriate Federal and State legislation, the Comprehensive Health Insurance Plan would offer to every American the same broad and balanced health protection through one of three major programs:

--Employee Health Insurance, covering most Americans and offered at their place of employment, with the cost to be shared by the employer and employee on a basis which would prevent excessive burdens on either;

--Assisted Health Insurance, covering low-income persons, and persons who would be ineligible for the other two programs, with Federal and State government paying those costs beyond the means of the individual who is insured; and,

--An improved Medicare Plan, covering those 65 and over and offered through a Medicare system that is modified to include additional, needed benefits. One of these three plans would be available to every American, but for everyone, participation in the program would be voluntary.

The benefits offered by the three plans would be identical for all Americans, regardless of age or income. Benefits would be provided for: --hospital care; --physicians' care in and out of the hospital; --prescription and life-saving drugs; --laboratory tests and X-rays; --medical devices; --ambulance services; and, --other ancillary health care.

There would be no exclusions of coverage based on the nature of the illness. For example, a person with heart disease would qualify for benefits as would a person with kidney disease.

In addition, CHIP would cover treatment for mental illness, alcoholism and drug addiction, whether that treatment were provided in hospitals and physicians' offices or in community based settings.

Certain nursing home services and other convalescent services would also be covered. For example, home health services would be covered so that long and costly stays in nursing homes could be averted where possible.

The health needs of children would come in for special attention, since many conditions, if detected in childhood, can be prevented from causing lifelong disability and learning handicaps. Included in these services for children would be: --preventive care up to age six; --eye examinations; --hearing examinations; and, --regular dental care up to age 13.

Under the Comprehensive Health Insurance Plan, a doctor's decisions could be based on the health care needs of his patients, not on health insurance coverage. This difference is essential for quality care.

Every American participating in the program would be insured for catastrophic illnesses that can eat away savings and plunge individuals and families into hopeless debt for years. No family would ever have annual out-of-pocket expenses for covered health services in excess of $1,500, and low-income families would face substantially smaller expenses.

As part of this program, every American who participates in the program would receive a Health-card when the plan goes into effect in his State. This card, similar to a credit card, would be honored by hospitals, nursing homes, emergency rooms, doctors, and clinics across the country. This card could also be used to identify information on blood type and sensitivity to particular drugs-information which might be important in an emergency.

Bills for the services paid for with the Health-card would be sent to the insurance carrier who would reimburse the provider of the care for covered services, then bill the patient for his share, if any.

The entire program would become effective in 1976, assuming that the plan is promptly enacted by the Congress.

HOW EMPLOYEE HEALTH INSURANCE WOULD WORK

Every employer would be required to offer all full-time employees the Comprehensive Health Insurance Plan. Additional benefits could then be added by mutual agreement. The insurance plan would be jointly financed, with employers paying 65 percent of the premium for the first three years of the plan, and 75 percent thereafter. Employees would pay the balance of the premiums. Temporary Federal subsidies would be used to ease the initial burden on employers who face significant cost increases.

Individuals covered by the plan would pay the first $150 in annual medical expenses. A separate $50 deductible provision would apply for out-patient drugs. There would be a maximum of three medical deductibles per family.

After satisfying this deductible limit, an enrollee would then pay for 25 percent of additional bills. However, $1,500 per year would be the absolute dollar limit on any family's medical expenses for covered services in any one year.

As an interim measure, the Medicaid program would be continued to meet certain needs, primarily long-term institutional care. I do not consider our current approach to long-term care desirable because it can lead to overemphasis on institutional as opposed to home care. The Secretary of Health, Education, and Welfare has undertaken a thorough study of the appropriate institutional services which should be included in health insurance and other programs and will report his findings to me.

IMPROVING MEDICARE

The Medicare program now provides medical protection for over 23 million older Americans. Medicare, however, does not cover outpatient drugs, nor does it limit total out-of-pocket costs. It is still possible for an elderly person to be financially devastated by a lengthy illness even with Medicare coverage. I therefore propose that Medicare's benefits be improved so that Medicare would provide the same benefits offered to other Americans under Employee Health Insurance and Assisted Health Insurance.

Any person 65 or over, eligible to receive Medicare payments, would ordinarily, under my modified Medicare plan, pay the first $100 for care received during a year, and the first $50 toward outpatient drugs. He or she would also pay 20 percent of any bills above the deductible limit. But in no case would any Medicare beneficiary have to pay more than $750 in out-of-pocket costs. The premiums and cost sharing for those with low incomes would be reduced, with public funds making up the difference.

The current program of Medicare for the disabled would be replaced. Those now in the Medicare for the disabled plan would be eligible for Assisted Health Insurance, which would provide better coverage for those with high medical costs and low incomes.

Premiums for most people under the new Medicare program would be roughly equal to that which is now payable under Part B of Medicare--the Supplementary Medical Insurance program.

HOW ASSISTED HEALTH INSURANCE WOULD WORK

The program of Assisted Health Insurance is designed to cover everyone not offered coverage under Employee Health Insurance or Medicare, including the unemployed, the disabled, the self-employed, and those with low incomes. In addition, persons with higher incomes could also obtain Assisted Health Insurance if they cannot otherwise get coverage at reasonable rates. Included in this latter group might be persons whose health status or type of work puts them in high-risk insurance categories.

Assisted Health Insurance would thus fill many of the gaps in our present health insurance system and would ensure that for the first time in our Nation's history, all Americans would have financial access to health protection regardless of income or circumstances.

A principal feature of Assisted Health Insurance is that it relates premiums and out-of-pocket expenses to the income of the person or family enrolled. Working families with incomes of up to $5,000, for instance, would pay no premiums at all. Deductibles, co-insurance, and maximum liability would all be pegged to income levels.

Assisted Health Insurance would replace State-run Medicaid for most services. Unlike Medicaid, where benefits vary in each State, this plan would establish uniform benefit and eligibility standards for all low-income persons. It would also eliminate artificial barriers to enrollment or access to health care.

COSTS OF COMPREHENSIVE HEALTH INSURANCE

When fully effective, the total new costs of CHIP to the Federal and State governments would be about $6.9 billion with an additional small amount for transitional assistance for small and low wage employers:

--The Federal Government would add about $5.9 billion over the cost of continuing existing programs to finance health care for low-income or high-risk persons.

--State governments would add about $1.0 billion over existing Medicaid spending for the same purpose, though these added costs would be largely, if not wholly offset by reduced State and local budgets for direct provision of services.

--The Federal Government would provide assistance to small and low wage employers which would initially cost about $450 million but be phased out over five years.

For the average American family, what all of these figures reduce to is simply this:

--The national average family cost for health insurance premiums each year under Employee Health Insurance would be about $150; the employer would pay approximately $450 for each employee who participates in the plan.

--Additional family costs for medical care would vary according to need and use, but in no case would a family have to pay more than $1,500 in any one year for covered services.

--No additional taxes would be needed to pay for the cost of CHIP. The Federal funds needed to pay for this plan could all be drawn from revenues that would be generated by the present tax structure. I am opposed to any comprehensive health plan which requires new taxes.

MAKING THE HEALTH CARE SYSTEM WORK BETTER

Any program to finance health care for the Nation must take close account of two critical and related problems--cost and quality.

When Medicare and Medicaid went into effect, medical prices jumped almost twice as fast as living costs in general in the next five years. These programs increased demand without increasing supply proportionately and higher costs resulted.

This escalation of medical prices must not recur when the Comprehensive Health Insurance Plan goes into effect. One way to prevent an escalation is to increase the supply of physicians, which is now taking place at a rapid rate. Since 1965, the number of first-year enrollments in medical schools has increased 55 percent. By 1980, the Nation should have over 440,000 physicians, or roughly one-third more than today. We are also taking steps to train persons in allied health occupations, who can extend the services of the physician.

With these and other efforts already underway, the Nation's health manpower supply will be able to meet the additional demands that will be placed on it.

Other measures have also been taken to contain medical prices. Under the New Economic Policy, hospital cost increases have been cut almost in half from their post-Medicare highs, and the rate of increase in physician fees has slowed substantially. It is extremely important that these successes be continued as we move toward our goal of comprehensive health insurance protection for all Americans. I will, therefore, recommend to the Congress that the Cost of Living Council's authority to control medical care costs be extended.

To contain medical costs effectively over the long-haul, however, basic reforms in the financing and delivery of care are also needed. We need a system with built-in incentives that operates more efficiently and reduces the losses from waste and duplication of effort. Everyone pays for this inefficiency through their health premiums and medical bills.

The measure I am recommending today therefore contains a number of proposals designed to contain costs, improve the efficiency of the system and assure quality health care. These proposals include:

1. HEALTH MAINTENANCE ORGANIZATIONS (HMO'S)

On December 29, 1973, I signed into law legislation designed to stimulate, through Federal aid, the establishment of prepaid comprehensive care organizations. HMO's have proved an effective means for delivering health care and the CHIP plan requires that they be offered as an option for the individual and the family as soon as they become available. This would encourage more freedom of choice for both patients and providers, while fostering diversity in our medical care delivery system.

2. PROFESSIONAL STANDARDS REVIEW ORGANIZATIONS (PSRO'S)

I also contemplate in my proposal a provision that would place health services provided under CHIP under the review of Professional Standards Review Organizations. These PSRO's would be charged with maintaining high standards of care and reducing needless hospitalization. Operated 'by groups of private physicians, professional review organizations can do much to ensure quality care while helping to bring about significant savings in health costs.

3. MORE BALANCED GROWTH IN HEALTH FACILITIES

Another provision of this legislation would call on the States to review building plans for hospitals, nursing homes and other health facilities. Existing health insurance has overemphasized the placement of patients in hospitals and nursing homes. Under this artificial stimulus, institutions have felt impelled to keep adding bed space. This has produced a growth of almost 75 percent in the number of hospital beds in the last twenty years, so that now we have a surplus of beds in many places and a poor mix of facilities in others. Under the legislation I am submitting, States can begin remedying this costly imbalance.

4. STATE ROLE

Another important provision of this legislation calls on the States to review the operation of health insurance carriers within their jurisdiction. The States would approve specific plans, oversee rates, ensure adequate disclosure, require an annual audit and take other appropriate measures. For health care providers, the States would assure fair reimbursement for physician services, drugs and institutional services, including a prospective reimbursement system for hospitals.

A number of States have shown that an effective job can be done in containing costs. Under my proposal all States would have an incentive to do the same. Only with effective cost control measures can States ensure that the citizens receive the increased health care they need and at rates they can afford. Failure on the part of States to enact the necessary authorities would prevent them from receiving any Federal support of their State-administered health assistance plan.

MAINTAINING A PRIVATE ENTERPRISE APPROACH

My proposed plan differs sharply with several of the other health insurance plans which have been prominently discussed. The primary difference is that my proposal would rely extensively on private insurers.

Any insurance company which could offer those benefits would be a potential supplier. Because private employers would have to provide certain basic benefits to their employees, they would have an incentive to seek out the best insurance company proposals and insurance companies would have an incentive to offer their plans at the lowest possible prices. If, on the other hand, the Government were to act as the insurer, there would be no competition and little incentive to hold down costs.

There is a huge reservoir of talent and skill in administering and designing health plans within the private sector. That pool of talent should be put to work.

It is also important to understand that the CHIP plan preserves basic freedoms for both the patient and doctor. The patient would continue to have a freedom of choice between doctors. The doctors would continue to work for their patients, not the Federal Government. By contrast, some of the national health plans that have been proposed in the Congress would place the entire health system under the heavy hand of the Federal Government, would add considerably to our tax burdens, and would threaten to destroy the entire system of medical care that has been so carefully built in America.

I firmly believe we should capitalize on the skills and facilities already in place, not replace them and start from scratch with a huge Federal bureaucracy to add to the ones we already have.

COMPREHENSIVE HEALTH INSURANCE PLAN--A PARTNERSHIP EFFORT

No program will work unless people want it to work. Everyone must have a stake in the process.

This Comprehensive Health Insurance Plan has been designed so that everyone involved would have both a stake in making it work and a role to play in the process consumer, provider, health insurance carrier, the States and the Federal Government. It is a partnership program in every sense.

By sharing costs, consumers would have a direct economic stake in choosing and using their community's health resources wisely and prudently. They would be assisted by requirements that physicians and other providers of care make available to patients full information on fees, hours of operation and other matters affecting the qualifications of providers. But they would not have to go it alone either: doctors, hospitals and other providers of care would also have a direct stake in making the Comprehensive Health Insurance Plan work. This program has been designed to relieve them of much of the red tape, confusion and delays in reimbursement that plague them under the bewildering assortment of public and private financing systems that now exist. Health-cards would relieve them of troublesome bookkeeping. Hospitals could be hospitals, not bill collecting agencies.

CONCLUSION

Comprehensive health insurance is an idea whose time has come in America.

There has long been a need to assure every American financial access to high quality health care. As medical costs go up, that need grows more pressing.

Now, for the first time, we have not just the need but the will to get this job done. There is widespread support in the Congress and in the Nation for some form of comprehensive health insurance.

Surely if we have the will, 1974 should also be the year that we find the way.

The plan that I am proposing today is, I believe, the very best way. Improvements can be made in it, of course, and the Administration stands ready to work with the Congress, the medical profession, and others in making those changes.

But let us not be led to an extreme program that would place the entire health care system under the dominion of social planners in Washington.

Let us continue to have doctors who work for their patients, not for the Federal Government. Let us build upon the strengths of the medical system we have now, not destroy it.

Indeed, let us act sensibly. And let us act now--in 1974--to assure all Americans financial access to high quality medical care.

RICHARD NIXON

The White House,

February 6, 1974.

Note: On the same day, the White House released a fact sheet and the transcript of a news briefing on the message by Secretary of Health, Education, and Welfare Caspar W. Weinberger.

Citation: John T. Woolley and Gerhard Peters, The American Presidency Project [online]. Santa Barbara, CA. Available from World Wide Web: http://www.presidency.ucsb.edu/ws/?pid=4337

ABOOUT THE AUTHOR

Genrich Krasko was born and educated in Russia. In December 1977 he and his family (wife and teenage son) immigrated to Israel. They moved to the U.S. in 1980.

After leaving Russia, Krasko, a Ph.D. in physics of metals, did research and taught physics at universities in Israel, Germany, and the U.S. The last 11 years of his career as a physicist he was doing research in the U.S. Army Research Laboratory, from which he retired in 1999.

In 1996, while researching the strength of metals, Krasko finished writing a non-fiction book titled *This Unbearable Boredom of Being: A Crisis of Meaning in America*, to which Viktor Frankl, the great Austrian psychologist, psychiatrist, and author of the internationally acclaimed book *Man's Search for Meaning*, wrote a foreword. The book was published in 2004.

His second book, a novel in e-mails with a science-fiction twist (written in 2003-2004), can be found on Amazon.com in a Kindle format.

The book you just finished reading is his third book.

Krasko has a website, *www.SayNoToBoredom.com*, dedicated to Viktor Frankl's Centennial (2005). It contains additional information on his first book and a number of unpublished essays, among them: "The Battered First Amendment – The Abandoned Ninth,"(1997), "Training or Education? America's Cultural and Existential Dilemma"(2001), "Will the Internet Kill the Book?"(2007), "Some Thoughts on Education"(2010), and "Does Life Have Purpose and Meaning? An Imaginary Conversation With Teenagers" (2012).

Genrich Krasko lives with his wife, Zeya, in Peabody, MA.

Who Cares about Health Care?

REFERENCES

Introduction

[1] *All Amendments to the United States Constitution:*
http://www1.umn.edu/humanrts/education/all_amendments_usconst.htm
[2] Daniel Farber. (April 27, 2007).*The 'Silent' Ninth Amendment Gives Americans Rights They Don't Know They Have*:
http://www.alternet.org/story/50404/the_'silent'_ninth_amendment_gives_americans _rights_they_don't_know_they_have
[3] *Poll finds Americans split by political party over whether socialized medicine better or worse than current system:* http://www.hsph.harvard.edu/news/press-releases/poll-americans-split-by-political-party-over-socialized-medicine/
[4] *Otto von Bismarck*: http://en.wikipedia.org/wiki/Otto_von_Bismarck
[5] *Health Insurance Act of 1883*:
http://imagine.wikia.com/wiki/Health_Insurance_Act_of_1883
[6] *Medieval Guilds and social security*: http://www.aeans.org/articles/guilds.shtml
[7] George Rosen. *A History of Public Health Care*. The Johns Hopkins University Press, 1993, pp. 22-24.
[8] Richard Nixon's *Special Message to the Congress* of 6 February 1974:
http://www.presidency.ucsb.edu/ws/index.php?pid=3757#axzz1Ootw4IFd

History of Health Care in America

[1] *Flexner Report*: http://en.wikipedia.org/wiki/Flexner_Report
[2] Melissa Thomasson, *Health Insurance in the United States*.
http://eh.net/encyclopedia/health-insurance-in-the-united-states/
[3] Karen S. Palmer. *A Brief History: Universal Health Care Efforts in the US*.
http://www.pnhp.org/facts/a_brief_history_universal_health_care_efforts_in_the_us. php?page=all
[4] Wasley, Terree P. *Health Care In The Twentieth Century: A History of Government Interference And Protection*: http://www.freepatentsonline.com/article/business-economics/13834930.html
[5] *Kaiser Permanente. History*: http://share.kaiserpermanente.org/article/history-of-kaiser-permanente
[6] *State of the Union and Health Care: 100 Years of Good Intentions:*
http://www.medscape.com/features/slideshow/sotu?src=mp&spon=34
[7] *The New Deal*: http://en.wikipedia.org/wiki/The_New_Deal
[8] Franklin D. Roosevelt. *Second Bill of Rights*:
http://www.presidency.ucsb.edu/ws/index.php?pid=16518#axzz1lLxzOaNK
[9] *Harry S. Truman's 1948 State of the Union Address*:
http://www.trumanlibrary.org/whistlestop/tap/1748.htm

[10] *Dwight D. Eisenhower's 1956 State of the Union Address*:
http://www.pbs.org/wgbh/americanexperience/features/primary-
resources/eisenhower-state56/?flavour=mobile

[11] Igor Vosky. Jul.29, 2009. *Republicans Opposed Medicare In 1960s* :
http://thinkprogress.org/health/2009/07/29/170887/medicare-44/?mobile=nc

[12] *Great Society* http://en.wikipedia.org/wiki/Great_Society

[13] *Social Security Act of 1965:*
http://www.multilingualarchive.com/ma/enwiki/en/Social_Security_Act_of_1965

[14] *The Medicaid* http://en.wikipedia.org/wiki/Medicade

[15] Health care Financing review/winter 2005-2006. *Medicare and Medicaid history milestones:* https://www.cms.gov/Health careFinancingReview/downloads/05-06Winpg1.pdf

[16] *Richard Nixon's 34th Special Message to the Congress Proposing a Comprehensive Health Insurance Plan*:
http://www.presidency.ucsb.edu/ws/?pid=4337

[17] Ben Stein. Mar. 25, 2010. *Giving Nixon His Due on Health care Reform*:
http://www.aolnews.com/2010/03/25/opinion-giving-nixon-his-due-on-health-care-reform/

[18] *Jimmy Carter's Health care Legislation Message to the Congress:*
http://www.presidency.ucsb.edu/ws/index.php?pid=7401

[19] *Jimmy Carter blasts Ted Kennedy in '60 Minutes' interview* (16 Sent. 2010):
http://www.cbsnews.com/video/watch/?id=6872807n

[20] Timothy Stanley. *Memo to Jimmy Carter: Ted Kennedy Didn't Sabotage Health care Reform*: http://hnn.us/articles/131473.html

[21] Associated press. *Kennedy Regretted Having killed Nixon's reform*:
http://www.kaiserhealthnews.org/Daily-Reports/2010/September/17/Carter-and-Kennedy.aspx

[22] *Ronald Reagan Speaks Out Against Socialized Medicine:*
http://www.youtube.com/watch?v=fRdLpem-AAs

[23] Michael L. Millenson, Feb. 16, 2010. *Health Reform that Scares Both Parties*:
http://www.kaiserhealthnews.org/Columns/2010/February/021610Millenson.aspx

[24] M. Grealy. Jul. 1998. *Overview of the Medicare Catastrophic Coverage Act of 1988 and its impact on health-care delivery:*
http://www.ncbi.nlm.nih.gov/pubmed/2672805

[25] *George H. W. Bush's State of the Union Address* (28 January, 1992):
http://www.infoplease.com/t/hist/state-of-the-union/205.html

[26] *Clinton Health care Plan of 1993*:
http://en.wikipedia.org/wiki/Clinton_health_care_plan_of_1993

[27] PBS. *A Detailed Timeline of the Health care Debate:*
http://www.democraticunderground.com/discuss/duboard.php?az=view_all&address=389x4633336

[28] Paul Starr Paul Starr, *What Happened to Health care Reform?* The American Prospect no. 20 (Winter 1995): 20-31. http://www.princeton.edu/~starr/20starr.html

[29] President Clinton. *1995 State of the Union Address*:
http://www.washingtonpost.com/wp-srv/politics/special/states/docs/sou95.htm

[30]President Clinton. *1999 State of the Union Address:*
http://www.washingtonpost.com/wp-srv/politics/special/states/docs/sou99.htm
[31] *George W. Bush's Health-Care Plans:*
 http://www.webmd.com/medicare/features/george-w-bushs-health-care-plans
[32] *Medicare Part D coverage gap:*
http://en.wikipedia.org/wiki/Medicare_Part_D_coverage_gap
[33] *Bush Promotes Health Savings Accounts:* http://www.washingtonpost.com/wp-dyn/articles/A39782-2005Jan26.html
[34] *H.R. 525. Congressional Budget Office Estimate*:
http://www.thefreelibrary.com/Association+health+plan+legislation+introduced.+(H eadlines).(American...-a098977588
[35] *States Moving Toward Comprehensive Health care Reform:*
http://www.kff.org/uninsured/kcmu_statehealthreform.cfm

Health Care in the World

Canada

[1] Laura Steiner, *Structure and History of Canadian Health care*:
https://suite101.com/a/structure-and-history-of-canadian-health care-a140671
[2] Karen S. Palmer; Talk in 1999 PNNP Meeting. *A Brief History: Universal Health care Efforts in the U.S.*: http://www.pnhp.org/facts/a-brief-history-universal-health-care-efforts-in-the-us
[3] *Canadian Health care Five Principles*: http://www.canadian-health care.org/page2.html
[4] Canadian Revenue Agency. *2014 Income Tax Rates for Individuals*:
http://www.cra-arc.gc.ca/tx/ndvdls/fq/txrts-eng.html
[5] The Commonwealth Fund. *International Profiles of Health care Systems, 2012:*
http://www.commonwealthfund.org/~/media/Files/Publications/Fund%20Report/201 2/Nov/1645_Squires_intl_profiles_hlt_care_systems_2012.pdf
[6] *Poor, sick and uninsured Canadians least likely to afford prescription drug*s:
http://www.thestar.com/news/gta/2012/01/16/poor_sick_and_uninsured_canadians_l east_likely_to_afford_prescription_drugs.html
[7] *Public vs. Private:* http://www.cbc.ca/news/background/health care/public_vs_private.html
[8] *OECD Health Data 2012*: http://www.oecd.org/health/health-systems/oecdhealthdata2012.htm
[9] Angie Mohr, May 14, 2012. *Maternity Leave Basics: Canada vs. the U.S.*:
http://www.investopedia.com/financial-edge/0512/maternity-leave-basics-canada-vs.-the-u.s..aspx#axzz27he3lWQ6
[10] Ken McNaughton, *Long-Term Care Insurance in Canada*:
http://www.senioryears.com/longtermcare.html
[11] *Ontario Nursing Homes:* http://www.nursinghomeratings.ca/understand-the-nursing-home-system/ontario
[12] *Healthy Canadians. A Federal Report On Comparable Health Indicators, 2010*:
 http://www.hc-sc.gc.ca/hcs-sss/pubs/system-regime/2010-fed-comp-indicat/index-eng.php#t18

[13] *Comparison of Health care Systems in Canada and the United States,* August, 2013: http://www.peacebridgehealth care.com/blog/10/comparison-of-health-care-systems-in-canada-and-the-united-states.aspx

[14] Jason Shafrin (Oct 2, 2007), *Health care System Grudge Match: Canada vs. U.S.:* http://health care-economist.com/2007/10/02/health-care-system-grudge-match-canada-vs-us/

[15] *CIA The World Factbook:* https://www.cia.gov/library/publications/the-world-factbook/rankorder/2091rank.html

[16]*Health care In Canada vs Health care In The United States. Sec. 4.4: Malpractice litigations*: http://www.diffen.com/difference/Health care_In_Canada_vs_Health care_In_The_United_States#Malpractice_litigation

[17] Series of AMA proposal for Reform: *Administrative costs of health care coverage* : http://academic.udayton.edu/lawrenceulrich/315Articles/AMAadmincosts.pdf

[18] Health Affairs. Dante Morra, et al. (May 2014). *US Physician Practices Versus Canadians: Spending Nearly Four Times As Much Money Interacting With Payers:* http://content.healthaffairs.org/content/30/8/1443

France

[1] *Being Sick in France*: http://www.understandfrance.org/Paris/Sick.html

[2] Rebecca Leung (June 25, 2005). *France: Less Work, More Time Off.* : http://www.cbsnews.com/stories/2005/06/27/60II/main704571.shtml?tag=contentMain;contentBody

[3] Niall McKay. *Paying With Plastic: How It Works In The Rest Of The World*: http://www.pbs.org/wgbh/pages/frontline/shows/credit/more/world.html

[4] *The French lesson in Health care:* http://www.businessweek.com/magazine/content/07_28/b4042070.htm

[5] David Hamilton. June 1, 2011. *The French health care system is the best in the world*: http://theragblog.blogspot.com/2011/06/david-p-hamilton-french-health care-is.html

[6] A comprehensive review of the French Social Security System can be found in this 2010 document: *http://www.cleiss.fr/docs/regimes/regime_france/an_index.html*

[7] *Summary of Social Security and Private Employee benefits. France 2012*: http://www.igpinfo.com/igpinfo/public_documents/ss_summaries/France.pdf

[8] *The Holocaust: The French Vichy Regime:* http://www.jewishvirtuallibrary.org/jsource/Holocaust/VichyRegime.html

[9] *Health Reform – France III:* http://abriefhistory.org/?tag=france

[10] OECD Health Data 2012 - Frequently Requested Data: http://www.oecd.org/health/health-systems/oecdhealthdata2012-frequentlyrequesteddata.htm

[11] *Payroll Deductions. The Table is based on the numbers from* (2014): http://www.french-property.com/guides/france/finance-taxation/taxation/social-security/social-welfare-levy/ and http://www.cleiss.fr/docs/regimes/regime_france/an_a2.html

[12] *French Income Tax Rates for 2014*: http://www.french-property.com/news/tax_france/income_tax_bands_2014/

[13] *France VAT (Jan. 1,2014)*: http://www.tmf-vat.com/vat/france-vat.html

[14] À Aimer. Getting Sick, Part Four:
http://foreignparts.typepad.com/foreign_parts/2009/10/à-aimer-getting-sick-part-four.html

[15] *Cost Sharing for Health care: France, Germany, and Switzerland*:
http://www.kff.org/insurance/upload/7852.pdf

[16] *The Commonwealth Fund 2013 International Health Policy Survey in Eleven Countries:*
http://www.commonwealthfund.org/~/media/Files/Publications/In%20the%20Literature/2013/Nov/PDF_Schoen_2013_IHP_survey_chartpack_final.pdf

[17] Standard Physicians' Fees: *http://en.wikipedia.org/wiki/Health_in_France*

[18] *Hospital Treatment in France:* http://www.french-property.com/guides/france/public-services/health/receiving-treatment/hospital-treatment/

[19] *Having a Baby in France:* http://riviera.angloinfo.com/information/health care/pregnancy-birth/

[20] Nursery Schools in France: http://www.frenchentree.com/fe-education/DisplayArticle.asp?ID=71

[21] *How Does U.S. Long-Term Care Stack Up Against the Rest of the World?:*
http://www.kaiserhealthnews.org/Columns/2010/January/011910Gleckman.aspx

[22] Christophe Courbage & Nolwenn Roudaut (2010). *On Insurance for Long Term Care in France:* http://www.cesifo-group.de/portal/page/portal/DocBase_Content/ZS/ZS-CESifo_DICE_Report/zs-dice-2010/zs-dice-2010-2/dicereport210-forum4.pdf

[23] *Emergency Medical Services in France:*
http://en.wikipedia.org/wiki/Emergency_medical_services_in_France

[24] *French Health Insurance Card - Carte Vitale:* http://www.french-property.com/guides/france/public-services/health/health-card/

[25] Victor G. Rodwin &Simone Sandier. *Health care Under French National Health Insurance:* http://www.nyu.edu/projects/rodwin/french.html

Germany

[1] Marc S. Micozzi M.D. Nov 01, 1993. *National Health care: Medicine in Germany, 1918–1945*: http://www.fee.org/the_freeman/detail/national-health-care-medicine-in-germany-1918-1945

[2] Dr. Robert N. Proctor, *Dimensions*, Vol 10, No 2, 1996, *Nazi Medicine and Public Health Policy*: http://www.adl.org/braun/dim_14_1_nazi_med.asp

[3] Health Insurance Options in Germany – 2013:
http://www.howtogermany.com/pages/healthinsurance2.html

[4] *Frequently Asked Questions About Health care Coverage in Germany*:
http://americanviewsabroad.org/FAQs_about_health care_in_Germany_v4.pdf

[5] *Getting Public Health Insurance When Self-Employed:*
http://www.toytowngermany.com/lofi/index.php/t88321-15.html

[6] *Germany: Self-Employed Workers:*
http://www.eurofound.europa.eu/comparative/tn0801018s/de0801019q.htm

Who Cares about Health Care?

[7] *Health care in Germany:* http://www.civitas.org.uk/pubs/bb3Germany.php

[8] Augurzky, Boris, et al. *Copayments in the German Health System. Does it Work?* :http://www.econstor.eu/dspace/bitstream/10419/33970/1/530032120.pdf

[9] *Germany's New System of Parental Leave* (since 2007): http://www.janvonbroeckel.de/english/parental_leave.html

[10] *Fertility statistics:* http://epp.eurostat.ec.europa.eu/statistics_explained/index.php/Fertility_statistics

[11] *Early Childhood Education and Care in Germany:* http://www.tulane.edu/~rouxbee/soci626/germany/_pbaliga/early%20childhood%20 education%20and%20care.htm

[12] OECD 2011.Long-Term Health care in Germany: http://www.oecd.org/dataoecd/2/17/47908269.pdf

[13] Long-term care insurance in Germany: what can be learned from the first 15 years?: http://www.zes.uni-bremen.de/ccm/cms-service/stream/asset/?asset_id=3458356

[14] *Social Security Programs Throughout Europe, 2012*: http://www.ssa.gov/policy/docs/progdesc/ssptw/2012-2013/europe/germany.html

[15] *Unemployment insurance*: http://www.justlanded.com/english/Germany/Germany-Guide/Jobs/Unemployment-insurance

[16] *Emergency Medical Services in Germany:* http://en.wikipedia.org/wiki/Emergency_medical_services_in_Germany

[17] *Anglo-American vs. Franco-German Emergency Medical Services System*: http://www.ncbi.nlm.nih.gov/pubmed/14694898

[1] *Life After the Baby Boomers: Keynote Address by Phil Zarlengo at the OECD Forum 2011:* http://www.aarpinternational.org/resourcelibrary/resourcelibrary_show.htm?doc_id= 1588779

[2] AARP. *Much to Learn from German Long-Term Care System*: http://www2.prnewswire.com/cgi-bin/stories.pl?%20ACCT=104&STORY=/www/story/10-30-2007/0004693363&EDATE

Japan

[3] Japan's Experiences in Public Health and Medical Systems (March, 2005): http://jica-ri.jica.go.jp/IFIC_and_JBICI-Studies/english/publications/reports/study/topical/health/pdf/health_01.pdf

[4] The American Occupation and Reconstruction of Japan (1945-1952): http://history.state.gov/milestones/1945-1952/japan-reconstruction

[5] Tetsuo Fukawa. Public Health Insurance in Japan : http://unpan1.un.org/intradoc/groups/public/documents/APCITY/UNPAN020063.pdf

[6] Blaine Harden (Sept. 7, 2009). Japan's Health-Care System Has Many Advantages, but May Not Be Sustainable: http://www.washingtonpost.com/wp-dyn/content/article/2009/09/06/AR2009090601630.html

[7] Health and Welfare: http://www.japan-zone.com/new/welfare.shtml

[8] Jason Shafrin (April, 2008). Health care Around the World. Japan : http://health care-economist.com/2008/04/17/health-care-around-the-world-japan/

[9] Lawrence A. Starr (Oct. 30, 2011) Doctors in Japan: http://maxfavorit.ru/doctors-in-japan-vrach-v-yaponii.htm

[10] The Current Medical Education in the world: http://lib.tmd.ac.jp/jmd/5802/07_Nara.pdf

[11] Valuing Medical Schools in Japan: National versus Private Universities: http://www2.econ.osaka-u.ac.jp/library/global/dp/0602.pdf

[12] Jason Shafrin (June, 2010). International Health care Models: Japan: http://health care-economist.com/2010/06/21/international-health care-models-japan/

[13] Japan Considers Automatic Redress Plan for Victims of Medical Malpractice: http://www.malpracticeinsuranceagency.com/blog/japan-considers-automatic-redress-plan-for-victims-of-medical-malpractice/

[14] Pre-Hospital Care System in Japan: http://www.ncbi.nlm.nih.gov/pmc/articles/PMC2672269/

[15] Nicole Crawford. Japan's Maternity Leave Laws: http://www.ehow.com/list_5982920_japan_s-maternity-leave-laws.html; http://lang-8.com/33465/journals/194768

[16] Japan With Kids. Life at Japanese Public Daycare: http://www.tokyowithkids.com/fyi/hoikuen.html

[17] Menstrual leave: http://en.wikipedia.org/wiki/Menstrual_Leave#cite_note-8

[18] Japan Demographics Profile 2013: http://www.indexmundi.com/japan/demographics_profile.html

[19] Dementia in Japan: http://www2f.biglobe.ne.jp/~boke/dementiaj.htm

[20] Japan's Long-Term Care Insurance Programs: http://www.kaigo.gr.jp/JLCIhp.htm

[21] The Care of Older People in Japan: Myths and Realities of Family 'Care': http://www.historyandpolicy.org/papers/policy-paper-121.html

[22] Complementary and Alternative Medicine Guide: http://www.umm.edu/altmed/

United Kingdom

[1] *NHS - The United Kingdom's Health care System*: http://www.disabled-world.com/medical/health care/uk-health care/

[2] *National Health Service History:* http://www.nhshistory.net/shorthistory.htm

[3] *NHS Patients' Rights:* http://www.adviceguide.org.uk/index/your_family/health/nhs_patients_rights.htm#Seeingaconsultant

[4] Taxation in the United Kingdom: http://en.wikipedia.org/wiki/Taxation_in_the_United_Kingdom#Personal_taxes

[5] National Insurance: https://www.gov.uk/national-insurance

[6] *Interview: Nigel Hawkes (April 2008):* http://www.pbs.org/wgbh/pages/frontline/sickaroundtheworld/interviews/hawkes.html

[7] *Your Rights in the NHS. Guide to NHS Waiting Times:*
http://www.nhs.uk/choiceintheNHS/Rightsandpledges/Waitingtimes/Pages/Guide%2
0to%20waiting%20times.aspx

[8] *Operational Standards for the Cancer Waiting Times Commitments:*
http://www.aswcs.nhs.uk/main.cfm?type=cancerwaitingtimes#1

[9] *GP Earnings and Expenses 2011-2012* (Sept. 2013):
http://www.hscic.gov.uk/catalogue/PUB11702/gp-earn-ex-1112-rep.pdf

[10] Nobua Tara, et al. (2011) *The Current Medical Education System in the World:*
http://lib.tmd.ac.jp/jmd/5802/07_Nara.pdf

[11] Keir Stone-Brown (28 Oct. 2013). *Bleak financial outlook faced by medical
students:* http://student.bmj.com/student/view-article.html?id=sbmj.f6377

[12] Stephen Adams (Dec. 2010). *999 ambulance response time scrapped*:
http://www.telegraph.co.uk/health/healthnews/8209263/999-ambulance-response-
time-scrapped.html

[13] *Maternity Pay and Leave* (last updated 6 April 2014):
https://www.gov.uk/maternity-pay-leave/pay

[14]*Foundation Years: Sure Start Children's Centers* (2013-2014):
http://www.publications.parliament.uk/pa/cm201314/cmselect/cmeduc/364/364.pdf

[15] *The British Education System*:
http://www.learnenglish.de/culture/educationculture.htm

[16] *NHS Continuing Care:*
http://www.nhs.uk/CarersDirect/guide/practicalsupport/Pages/NHSContinuingCare.a
spx

[17] *Caring For Our Future. Consultation on Reforming What and How People Pay
For Their Care and Support* (p.13):
https://www.gov.uk/government/uploads/system/uploads/attachment_data/file/23939
3/CONSULTATION_CaringForOurFuture_acc.pdf

[18] *National Institute for Health and Care Excellence: Guidance:*
http://www.ncbi.nlm.nih.gov/books/NBK11822/

[1] *Of NICE and Men:* http://online.wsj.com/article/SB124692973435303415.html

[2] *Is Public Health care in the UK as Sick as Rightwing America Claims?:*
http://www.guardian.co.uk/society/2009/aug/11/nhs-sick-health care-reform

Israel

[3] *Vital Statistics: Latest Population Statistics for Israel. Jewish Virtual Library.*
January, 2014:
http://www.jewishvirtuallibrary.org/jsource/Society_&_Culture/newpop.html

[4] *Myths and Facts. A Guide to Arab-Israeli Conflict:*
http://www.jewishvirtuallibrary.org/jsource/myths3/MFroots.html
http://www.youtube.com/watch?v=XGYxLWUKwWo&feature=channel_video_title

[5] The Health care in Israel – A Historical Perspective:
http://www.mfa.gov.il/MFA/History/Modern%20History/Israel%20at%2050/The%2
0Health%20Care%20System%20in%20Israel-%20An%20Historical%20Pe

[6] Ziv Hellman (15/05/2010) *Health care for All*:
http://www.jpost.com/LandedPages/PrintArticle.aspx?id=175612
[7] Marty Peretz (20 May 2010) *Do You Want A Really Excellent Medical System?*
Live In Israel Or At Least Learn About "Health care For All" In The Jewish State.
http://calevbenyefuneh.blogspot.com/2010/05/do-you-want-really-excellent-
medical.html
[8] *Health care in Israel for U.S. Audiences*: http://www.prhi.org/docs/133-11-Israel-
Health care-US-Audiences-2-REP-ENG.pdf
[9] Rachel Missanholtz and Bruce Rozen (Jan.2011). *The Medical Workforce and*
Government-supported Medical Education in Israel:
http://brookdaleheb.jdc.org.il/_Uploads/PublicationsFiles/137-11-Workforce-and-
Medical-Education-6-REP-ENG.pdf
[10] *United Hatzalah*: http://www.israelrescue.org/index.php
[11] *TEDMED: How did volunteers save more than 40,000 lives in 3 minutes (each)*
last year? http://www.tedmed.com/talks/show?id=47048
[12] *What is Maternity Leave in Israel?*: http://tin.tv/site/article/אגעב/what-is-
maternity-leave-in-israel
[13] *Health Services in Israel – 4th Edition* (2011):
http://www.moia.gov.il/Publications/health_en.pdf
[14] *Pre-schools & Kindergartens in Israel*: http://www.anglo-
list.com/index.php?option=com_content&view=article&id=94&Itemid=146
[15] *Israel. Long-term Care*: http://www.oecd.org/dataoecd/61/0/47877779.pdf
[16] *Health Diplomacy: Peace Through Health*: http://susan-
blumenthal.org/about/affiliations/health-diplomacy-peace-through-health/
[17] *Increase in Palestinians Treated in Israeli Hospitals (2013)*:
http://www.algemeiner.com/2013/08/02/increase-in-palestinians-treated-in-israeli-
hospitals/
[18] Ebonne Ruffins (Feb. 1 2011). :
http://www.cnn.com/2011/WORLD/meast/02/01/cnnheroes.roth/index.html
[19] Medical Tourism:
http://www.goisrael.com/Tourism_Eng/Tourist%20Information/Discover%20Israel/
Pages/Medical%20Tourism.aspx
[20] Nefesh B'Nefesh: http://www.nbn.org.il

Obamacare

[1] *H.R. 3962 (111th): Preservation of Access to Care for Medicare Beneficiaries and*
Pension Relief Act of 2010: http://www.govtrack.us/congress/bills/111/hr3962/text
[2] *H.R.3962*: http://docs.house.gov/rules/health/111_ahcaa.pdf;
Public Law 111-118 – Mar. 23, 2010: http://www.gpo.gov/fdsys/pkg/PLAW-
111publ148/pdf/PLAW-111publ148.pdf
[3] *H.R. 4872. Health Care and Education Reconciliation Act of 2010*:
http://en.wikipedia.org/wiki/Health_Care_and_Education_Reconciliation_Act
[4] *A Guide to the Supreme Court's Affordable Care Act Decision*:
http://www.kff.org/healthreform/upload/8332.pdf

Who Cares about Health Care?

[5] *Kaiser Health Tracking Poll: April 2013*:
http://kff.org/health-reform/poll-finding/kaiser-health-tracking-poll-april-2013/
[6] *Take Health care Into Your Own Hands*: http://www.health care.gov/
[7] *ObamaCare Facts. Dispelling the Myths. How Does ObamaCare Work?*:
http://obamacarefacts.com/howdoes-obamacare-work.php
[8] *Summary of the Affordable Care Act*:
http://www.kff.org/healthreform/upload/8061.pdf; http://healthreform.kff.org
Summary of New Health Reform Law:
 http://www.kaiserfamilyfoundation.files.wordpress.com/2011/04/8061-021.pdf
The Affordable Health Act: Three Years Post-Enactment
http://kaiserfamilyfoundation.files.wordpress.com/2013/04/84291.pdf
[9] *NFIB; Health care Information You Need To Know*: http://www.nfib.com/business-resources/health care?gclid=CN2Jlc-FtbECFQff4Aod2DMAow
[10] *RAND Analysis:*
http://www.rand.org/content/dam/rand/pubs/research_briefs/2010/RAND_RB9504.pdf;
[11] A Guide to Real Costs and Consequences of the New Health care Law:
http://www.cato.org/pubs/wtpapers/BadMedicineWP.pdf
[12] *Updated Estimates for the Insurance Coverage Provisions of the Affordable Care Act (Jul. 2012)*: http://www.cbo.gov/sites/default/files/cbofiles/attachments/03-13-Coverage%20Estimates.pdf
http://www.cbo.gov/sites/default/files/cbofiles/attachments/43471-hr6079.pdf
[13] *What's Really in the Affordable Care Act*:
http://www.medscape.com/features/slideshow/bm-aca
[14] *Income, Poverty, and Health Insurance Coverage in the U.S, 2011*:
http://www.census.gov/prod/2012pubs/p60-243.pdf
[15] *America's 6 Million To 8 Million Uninsured Need Help With Health care Bills:*
http://www.businessword.com/index.php?/weblog/comments/2303/
[16] *Average Annual Premiums for Family Health Benefits*:
http://www.kff.org/insurance/092311nr.cfm
[17] *A closer look at the individual mandate:*
http://www.putnamwealthmanagement.com/a-closer-look-at-the-individual-mandate
[18] *Taxing the Uninsured: The Latest Estimates (2012)*:
http://taxfoundation.org/article/taxing-uninsured-latest-estimates#_ftnref8
[19] *Essential Health Benefits, Actuarial Value, and Accreditation Standards:*
http://www.health care.gov/news/factsheets/2012/11/ehb11202012a.html
[20] *How New Health Insurance Subsidies Will Work*:
http://money.usnews.com/money/blogs/the-best-life/2012/07/27/how-new-health-insurance-subsidies-will-work
[21] *Explaining Health care Reform: Questions About Insurance Subsidies*:
http://www.kff.org/healthreform/upload/7962-02.pdf
[22]*CBO: Obamacare to Cover Millions Fewer Than Before Supreme Court Decision:*
http://blog.heritage.org/2012/07/24/cbo-obamacare-to-cover-millions-fewer-than-before-supreme-court-decision/
[23] *Congressional Budget Office. Changes in Payments to Physicians*:
http://www.cbo.gov/doc.cfm?index=12240

[24] *Obamacare Timeline*: http://health care-coalition.org/timeline
[25] *Health care Reform Will Impact Long-Term Care*:
http://www.healthleadersmedia.com/page-1/LED-248406/Health care-Reform-Will-Impact-Longterm-Care
[26] *CLASS is Killed: But How Will We Pay for Long-Term Care Services?*:
http://www.forbes.com/sites/howardgleckman/2011/10/15/Class-Is-Killed-But-How-Will-We-Pay-For-Long-Term-Care-Services/
[27] *State progress on Essential Health Benefits*: http://www.statereforum.org/state-progress-on-essential-health-benefits
[28] *USPHS Commissioned Corps Ready Reserve Corps*:
http://www.usphs.gov/pdf/Usphs_Commissioned_Corps_Ready_Reserve_Corps_Fact_Sheet.pdf
[29] *H.R. 3962 Summary*: http://emptysuit.wordpress.com/2009/10/29/h-r-3962-summary/
[30] *Progress Report on The Affordable Care Act*:
http://www.ccconsultingllc.com/progress-report-on-the-affordable-care-act/
[31] *The Patient Protection and Affordable Care Act (PPACA) Timeline*:
http://www.nfib.com/business-resources/health care/reform-timeline
[32] Medscape Oncology. Mar. 13, 2014. The ACA Open Enrollment at 2 Months: The View From Across the Country:
http://www.medscape.com/viewarticle/821858?nlid=51413_426&src=wnl_edit_medp_fmed&uac=46251FT&spon=34
[33] CNN Money. Mar. 19, 2014. Got Obamacare, Can't Find Doctors:
http://money.cnn.com/2014/03/19/news/economy/obamacare-doctors/index.html?hpt=hp_t2
[34] Massachusetts Health care Reform: Six Years Later (2012):
http://www.kff.org/healthreform/upload/8311.pdf
[35] Mass. Health Law Thrown a Curve by Obamacare:
http://www.bostonglobe.com/business/2012/11/11/employers-grapple-with-federal-health-care-reform/a4jGIKUOkLLU4SGzBh9myM/story.html
[36] States Moving Toward Comprehensive Health care Reform:
http://www.kff.org/uninsured/kcmu_statehealthreform.cf

Where Are We? America's Health Care Today

[1] *Are Patients in Universal Health Care Countries Less Satisfied?*
http://scienceblogs.com/denialism/2009/05/22/are-patients-in-universal-heal/
[2] *Health care Spending in the United States and Selected OECD Countries:*
http://www.kff.org/insurancCongressionale/snapshot/OECD042111.cfm
[3] *National Accounts at a Glance, 2013*: http://www.oecd-ilibrary.org/economics/national-accounts-at-a-glance-2013_na_glance-2013-en
[4] *Explaining High Health Care Spending in the United States: An International Comparison of Supply, Utilization, Prices, and Quality:*
http://www.commonwealthfund.org/~/media/Files/Publications/Issue%20Brief/2012/May/1595_Squires_explaining_high_hlt_care_spending_intl_brief.pdf

[5] *Putting Health Plans' Profits In Perspective:*
http://www.ahipcoverage.com/2011/03/03/putting-health-plans-profits-in-perspective/

[6] *Just How Profitable are Health care Insurers?:*
http://larrycheng.com/2010/03/08/just-how-profitable-are-health care-insurers/

[7] *Health Insurance Companies Rank #88 by Industry Profit Margin, Earning $100-200 on Average Per Policy:* http://mjperry.blogspot.com/2010/02/health-insurance-companies-rank-88-by.html

[8] *Marriott International Profit Margin:*
http://ycharts.com/companies/MAR/profit_margin

[9] Quoted in: *U.S. Health Care Spending In An International Context:*
http://content.healthaffairs.org/content/23/3/10.full

[10] *2013 Medscape Physician Compensation Report:*
http://www.medscape.com/features/slideshow/compensation/2013/public

[11] David Cutler, Ph.D., et al. *Reducing Administrative Costs and Improving the Health care System.*
N Engl J Med 2012; 367:1875-1878 November 15, 2012:
http://www.nejm.org/doi/full/10.1056/NEJMp1209711

[12] *Congressional Research Service. Medicare Financing and Expenditures. 2012:*
http://www.fas.org/sgp/crs/misc/R42640.pdf

[13] *Core Administrative Costs of Medicaid Plans Were 6.5% of Premiums in 2010:*
http://www.businesswire.com/news/home/20111014006050/en/Core-Administrative-Costs-Medicaid-Plans-6.5-Premiums

[14] *Richard Nixon's Special Message to the Congress of 6 February 1974:*
http://www.presidency.ucsb.edu/ws/index.php?pid=3757#axzz1Ootw4IFd

[15] Sarah Kliff, 16 Feb. 2010. *Health-Care Cards Could Help Heal a Broken System:*
http://www.thedailybeast.com/newsweek/2010/02/16/the-smart-set.html

[16] *Smart Card Alliance:* http://www.smartcardalliance.org/

[17] *Economic Stimulus Bill Mandates Electronic Health Records:*
http://www.forhealthfreedom.org/Publications/privacy/EconomicStimulusAndPrivacy4.html

[18] *Let's Pay Doctor:*
http://www.slate.com/articles/news_and_politics/prescriptions/2009/09/lets_pay_doctor.html

[19] *Physician Compensation Worldwide (2009):*
http://www.practicelink.com/magazine/vital-stats/physician-compensation-worldwide/print/

[20] *Estimating a Reasonable Patient Panel Size for Primary Care Physicians:*
http://www.annfammed.org/content/10/5/396.full

[21] *Association of American Medical Colleges:*
https://www.aamc.org/initiatives/fixdocshortage/

[22] Anthony Youn, M.D. (CNN News, March 16, 2012), *Why your waiter has an M.D:* http://thechart.blogs.cnn.com/2012/03/16/why-your-waiter-has-an-m-d/

[23] Alexandra Sowa McPartland. (The Atlantic, Sept.16, 2014). *Suicide and the Young Physician: http://www.theatlantic.com/health/archive/2014/09/suicide-and-the-young-physician/380253/*

[24] Louise B. Andrew, MD, JD, et al. (Medscape, Jul. 17, 2014). *Physician Suicide*: http://emedicine.medscape.com/article/806779-overview

[25] *Ensuring Access to Care in Medicaid Under Health Reform:* http://www.kff.org/healthreform/upload/8187.pdf

[26] Atul Gawande: *Better. A Surgeon's Notes on Performance (2008)* , p.87. Three other books: *Complications: A Surgeon's Notes on an Imperfect Science (2003), The Checklist Manifesto: How to Get Things Right (2011),* and *Being Mortal: Medicine and What Matters in the End (2014)*

[27] Carolyne F. Heffrich. Ph.D., et al. (2010). *The Cost of Defensive Medicine:* http://www.aaos.org/news/aaosnow/dec10/advocacy2.asp

[28] Michelle M. Mello, et al. *National Costs Of The Medical Liability System:* http://health.burgess.house.gov/UploadedFiles/Malpractice-Health_Affairs.pdf

[29] Stuart L. Weinstein, MD. *The Cost of Defensive Medicine:* http://www.aaos.org/news/aaosnow/nov08/managing7.asp

[30] Daphne Eviatar (Oct. 6, 2009). *Medical Malpractice Insurers' Profits Higher Than Nearly All Fortune 500 Companies:* http://washingtonindependent.com/62646/medical-malpractice-insurers-profits-higher-than-nearly-all-fortune-500-companies

[31] David A. Hyman and Charles Silver. *Medical Malpractice Litigation and Tart Reform:* http://iactprogram.com/wp-content/uploads/2011/09/Hyman_Silver1.pdf

[32] *Interview with Uwe Reinhardt and May Cheng* (Nov. 7, 2007): http://www.pbs.org/wgbh/pages/frontline/sickaroundtheworld/interviews/reinhardt.html

[33] *What Doctors Make and Why (2007):* http://query.nytimes.com/gst/fullpage.html?res=9B00EEDE163AF936A3575BC0A9619C8B63

[34] Michael D. Miller MD.(Feb. 5, 2013). *Health Spending: For What, To Whom, and Where It Is Heading:* http://www.healthpolcom.com/blog/2013/02/05/health-spending-for-what-to-whom-and-where-it-is-heading/

[35] *Best Care at Lower Cost: The Path to Continuously Learning Health care in America.* IOM Report, 6 Sept. 2012: http://www.iom.edu/Reports/2012/Best-Care-at-Lower-Cost-The-Path-to-Continuously-Learning-Health-Care-in-America.aspx.

[36] *How the U.S. Health-Care System Wastes $750 Billion Annually.* The Atlantic, 7 Sep. 2012: http://www.theatlantic.com/health/archive/2012/09/how-the-us-health-care-system-wastes-750-billion-annually/262106/

[37] *Health care Costs: A Primer Key Information On Health care Costs And Their Impact.* May, 2012: http://kaiserfamilyfoundation.files.wordpress.com/2013/01/7670-03.pdf

[38] Penelope Wang. (Dec. 12, 2012). *Cutting the high cost of end-of-life care:* http://money.cnn.com/2012/12/11/pf/end-of-life-care-duplicate-2.moneymag/index.html

[39] *Hospice Care Underused By Many Terminally Ill Patients, Study Finds:* http://web.med.harvard.edu/sites/RELEASES/html/052509_huskamp.html

[40] See an objective discussion of end-of-life controversy in a five-part article *Meet the Death Panel*: http://www.motherjones.com/politics/2010/07/health-care-rationing-death-panels?page=1; page=2; page=3; page=4; page=5.

[41] Marty Makary, MD. *Unaccountable. What Hospitals Won't Tell You and How Transparency Can Revolutionize Health care*. Bloomsbury Press, New York, 2012, p. 138.

[42] Richard A. Young, MD et al. (Sept. 13, 2011) *Who Will Have Health Insurance in the Future? An Updated Projection* :
http://www.annfammed.org/content/10/2/156.full.pdf

[43] *The Numbers Count: Mental Disorders in America:*
http://www.nimh.nih.gov/health/publications/the-numbers-count-mental-disorders-in-america/index.shtml#KesslerPrevalence

[44] *Mental Illness And Violence* (Jan. 2011):
http://www.health.harvard.edu/newsletters/Harvard_Mental_Health_Letter/2011/January/mental-illness-and-violence

[45] *Mental Illness and Homelessness* (Jul. 2009):
http://www.nationalhomeless.org/factsheets/Mental_Illness.pdf

[46] MacKenzie Kimball, (March 23, 2010). *Health care Reform Will Impact Long-Term Care:* http://www.healthleadersmedia.com/page-1/LED-248406/Health care-Reform-Will-Impact-Longterm-Care

[47] *CLASS is Killed: But How Will We Pay for Long-Term Care Services?:*
http://www.forbes.com/sites/howardgleckman/2011/10/15/class-is-killed-but-how-will-we-pay-for-long-term-care-services/

[48] *Alois Alzheimer:* http://www.alz.co.uk/alois-alzheime

[49] *2011 Alzheimer's Disease Facts and Figures*:
http://www.alz.org/downloads/Facts_Figures_2011.pdf

[50] Edward M. DeSimone I , Laura Viereck .(Jan. 2011): *Alzheimer's Disease Increasing Numbers, But No Cure:*
http://www.uspharmacist.com/content/c/26130/?t=alzheimer's_and_dementia;
Lancet, vol. 383, issue 9923, 29 March 2014. *Towards a Better Life With Alzheimer's Disease:* http://www.thelancet.com/journals/lancet/article/PIIS0140-6736(14)60548-1/fulltext?elsca1=ETOC-LANCET&elsca2=email&elsca3=E24A35F

[51] Elizabeth Landau, (Jul. 25,2011). *Alzheimer's: Early detection, risk factors are crucial:* http://www.cnn.com/2011/HEALTH/07/25/alzheimer.disease/index.html

[52] Patricia A. Boyle, PhD, et al. (May 2012). *Effect of Purpose in Life on the Relation Between Alzheimer Disease Pathologic Changes on Cognitive Function in Advanced Age*: http://archpsyc.jamanetwork.com/article.aspx?articleid=1151486

[53] Allison Gandey (March 03, 2010). *Purpose in Life May Reduce Alzheimer's Risk:*
http://www.medscape.com/viewarticle/717858

[54] *2013 Cost of Long Term Care by State:*
http://longtermcareinsurancepartner.com/long-term-care/2012-cost-of-long-term-care

[55] K. Gabriel Heiser. *How to Protect Your Family's Assets from Devastating Nursing Home Costs:* Medicaid Secrets. Lightning Source Incorporated, 6th edition, 2012;

[56] *CBO, March 2012. Updated Estimates for the Insurance Coverage Provisions of the Affordable Care Act*: http://cbo.gov/sites/default/files/cbofiles/attachments/03-13-Coverage%20Estimates.pdf

[57] *National Alzheimer's Project Act*: http://aspe.hhs.gov/daltcp/napa/

[58] *Obama Administration Presents National Plan To Fight Alzheimer's Disease:* http://www.nia.nih.gov/newsroom/2012/05/obama-administration-presents-national-plan-fight-alzheimers-disease

[59] *NIH. Estimates of Funding for Various Research, Condition, and Disease Categories (RCDC)*. March 7, 2014: http://report.nih.gov/categorical_spending.aspx

[60]Tanya Lewis (March 07, 2014). *President's Budget Would Double Funding for BRAIN Initiative:* http://www.livescience.com/43888-obama-budget-doubles-brain-funding.html

[61] Pam Belluck (NY Times, September 18, 2014. *Panel Urges Overhauling Health Care at End of Life: http://www.nytimes.com/2014/09/18/science/end-of-life-care-needs-sweeping-overhaul-panel-says.html?_r=0*

[62] Heidi Brown (May 05, 2009). *U.S. Maternity Leave Benefits Are Still Dismal:* http://www.forbes.com/2009/05/04/maternity-leave-laws-forbes-woman-wellbeing-pregnancy.html

[63] Sarah Fass (March 2009). Paid Leave in the States. *A Critical Support for Low-wage Workers and Their Families* : http://www.paidfamilyleave.org/pdf/PaidLeaveinStates.pdf

[64] Bernd Debusmann Jr (Feb 23, 2011). *U.S. Behind the World on Parental Leave: Report:* http://www.reuters.com/article/2011/02/23/us-usa-maternity-idUSTRE71M62P20110223

[65] *Parental Leave in the World:* http://en.wikipedia.org/wiki/Parental_leave#Benefits_in_a_selection_of_countries

[66] Dana Fenton (Oct. 2012). *Federal and State Maternity Benefits:* http://www.everydayfamily.com/federal-and-state-maternity-benefits/

[67] Rebecca Ray, et al. (Sept. 2008). *Parental Leave Policies in 21 Countries:* http://www.scribd.com/doc/5427460/Parental-Leave-Policies-in-21-Countries-Assessing-Generosity-and-Gender-Equality

[68] *2013 State Disability Insurance (SDI) Schedules:* https://www.vpaweb.com/about/pdf/SDI.pdf

[69] *President Obama Announces White House Council on Women and Girls* (March 2011): http://www.whitehouse.gov/the_press_office/President-Obama-Announces-White-House-Council-on-Women-and-Girls

[70] Maria Young. *Your Maternity Leave Plan of Action*: http://www.parents.com/pregnancy/my-life/maternity-paternity-leave/your-maternity-leave-plan-of-action/

[71] *Birth-18 Years & "Catch-up" Immunization Schedules* (2014): http://www.cdc.gov/vaccines/schedules/hcp/child-adolescent.html

[72] Saad B. Omer, M.B., B.S., Ph.D., M.P.H et al. (May 7, 2009). *Vaccine Refusal, Mandatory Immunization, and the Risks of Vaccine-Preventable Diseases:* http://www.nejm.org/doi/full/10.1056/NEJMsa0806477#t=articleTop

[73] *CDC. Some Common Misconceptions about vaccination and how to respond to them:* http://www.cdc.gov/vaccines/vac-gen/6mishome.htm

[74] Seth Mnookin (Oct 7, 2012). *Why So Many Parents Are Delaying or Skipping Vaccines*: http://www.parade.com/health/2012/10/07-why-so-many-parents-are-delaying-vaccines.html; http://www.parade.com/health/2012/10/07-why-so-many-parents-are-delaying-vaccines.html?index=2

[75] *Medicaid:* http://en.wikipedia.org/wiki/Medicaid

[76] *Medicare (United States):* http://en.wikipedia.org/wiki/Medicare_(United_States)

[77] CBO Updated Budget Projection: FY 2012 to 2022: http://www.cbo.gov/sites/default/files/cbofiles/attachments/March2012Baseline.pdf

[78] *ACA. Chapter 8 – Medicaid:* http://www.allhealth.org/sourcebookcontent.asp?CHID=71

[79] *Medicaid Enrollment : June 2012 Data Snapshot*: http://kaiserfamilyfoundation.files.wordpress.com/2013/08/8050-06-medicaid-enrollment.pdf

[80] *Medicaid Spending and Enrollment Detail for CBO's March 2012 Baseline:* http://www.cbo.gov/sites/default/files/cbofiles/attachments/43059_Medicaid.pdf

[81] *Premiums and Cost-Sharing in Medicaid:* http://kaiserfamilyfoundation.files.wordpress.com/2013/02/8416.pdf

[82] *Cost Sharing and Out of Pocket Costs. Medicaid:* http://www.medicaid.gov/Medicaid-CHIP-Program-Information/By-Topics/Cost-Sharing/Cost-Sharing-Out-of-Pocket-Costs.html

[83] *Medicare's Demographic Challenge—and the Urgent Need for Reform:* http://www.heritage.org/research/reports/2013/03/medicares-demographic-challenge-and-the-urgent-need-for-reform

[84] *Status of The Social Security And Medicare Programs. A Summary Of The 2013 Annual Reports:* http://www.ssa.gov/oact/trsum/index.html

[85] *FICA tax:* http://www.money-zine.com/Financial-Planning/Tax-Shelter/FICA-Tax/

[86] *Summary of Medicare Benefits and Cost-Sharing for 2014:* http://www.cahealthadvocates.org/basics/benefits-summary.html

[87] *Medicare Spending and Financing. FactSheet (Nov. 14, 2012):* http://www.kff.org/medicare/upload/7305-06.pdf

[88] *Medicare at a Glance:* http://kff.org/medicare/fact-sheet/medicare-at-a-glance-fact-sheet/

[89] Liz Kowalczyk (Aug. 25, 2013). *Status of Medicare patients can result in huge bills:* http://www.bostonglobe.com/lifestyle/health-wellness/2013/08/24/despite-long-hospital-stays-some-patients-never-admitted-leaving-them-with-huge-bills/UjD0YLmFZE2XMtBee6KveN/story.html?s_campaign=email_BG_TodaysHeadline

[90] *The Expanded and Improved Medicare For All Act (H.R. 676):* http://www.pnhp.org/publications/united-states-national-health-care-act-hr-676

[91] *A Summary of H.R. 676:* http://www.pnhp.org/news/2011/february/summary-hr-676-the-expanded-improved-medicare-for-all-act

How Are We Different?

[1]*Updated Estimates for the Insurance Coverage Provisions of the Affordable Care Act (March, 2012):*
http://www.cbo.gov/sites/default/files/cbofiles/attachments/03-13-Coverage%20Estimates.pdf

[2] *Medicaid Population:* http://www.medicaid.gov/Medicaid-CHIP-Program-Information/By-Population/By-Population.html

[1] *ObamaCare. Health Insurance Exchange*: http://obamacarefacts.com/obamacare-health-insurance-exchange.php

[2] *Health Affairs, Dec. 2010.* Quoted in:
http://theincidentaleconomist.com/wordpress/enough-with-the-wait-times-already/

[3] *Waiting Times. OECD Library:* http://www.oecd-ilibrary.org/docserver/download/8111101ec059.pdf?expires=1391721222&id=id&accname=guest&checksum=80CF4F18B9504B76909BFA66DE635FDD

[4] *What is the Independence at Home Act?:*
http://www.iahnow.com/IAHlegislation.htm

[5] *Why are the Israelis so Damn Happy?:*
http://www.thedailybeast.com/articles/2013/04/14/why-are-the-israelis-so-damn-happy.html

[6] *U.S. Health in International Perspective: Shorter Lives, Poorer Health:*
http://sites.nationalacademies.org/DBASSE/CPOP/US_Health_in_International_Perspective/index.htm#.UPMKo6WyPdk

[7] *U.S. Health care Spending: Comparison with Other OECD Countries*
http://assets.opencrs.com/rpts/RL34175_20070917.pdf

[8] *e-cigarettes: a moral quandary*:
http://www.thelancet.com/journals/lancet/article/PIIS0140-6736(13)61918-2/fulltext?elsca1=TLW_ETOC&elsca2=email&elsca3=E24A35F

[9] *Women and Smoking. An epidemic of smoking-related cancer and disease in women:* http://www.cancer.org/acs/groups/cid/documents/webcontent/002986-pdf.pdf

[10] David A. Squires (May, 2012). *Explaining High Health care Spending in the United States: An International Comparison of Supply, Utilization, Prices, and Quality*:
http://www.commonwealthfund.org/~/media/Files/Publications/Issue%20Brief/2012/May/1595_Squires_explaining_high_hlt_care_spending_intl_brief.pdf

[11] *Warning Signs of Stroke:*
http://www.stroke.org/site/PageServer?pagename=symp&s_subsrc=SEM_google_grant_Keyword%20Correlation_Symptoms%20Of%20Stroke_stroke%20symptoms_b_17770654790&utm_source=google&utm_medium=grant&utm_campaign=Keyword%20Correlation

[12] Andrea M. Braslavsky.WebMD Health News.(June 1, 2000). *Aspirin Taken Right After a Stroke May Prevent a Second One:*
http://www.webmd.com/stroke/news/20000601/aspirin-after-stroke-helps-prevent-another

[13] *Bloomberg's The World' Most Efficient Health care Systems:*
http://www.bloomberg.com/visual-data/best-and-worst/most-efficient-health-care-countries; *Bloomberg's The World' Healthiest Countries:*
http://images.businessweek.com/bloomberg/pdfs/worlds_healthiest_countries_V2.pdf

[14] *WHO Health care Ranking by Eight Measures:*
http://www.photius.com/rankings/world_health_systems.html

[15] *President's Budget Would Double Funding for BRAIN Initiative:*
http://www.livescience.com/43888-obama-budget-doubles-brain-funding.html

[16] Megan Mcardle (Mar 6, 2012) *France and U.S. Health care: Twins Separated at Birth?* http://www.theatlantic.com/business/archive/2012/03/france-and-us-health-care-twins-separated-at-birth/254033/

[17] *Health care Under French National Health Insurance:*
http://www.nyu.edu/projects/rodwin/french.html

[18] *International Federation of Health Plans. 2012 Comparative Price Report;*
http://www.ifhp.com/documents/2012iFHPPriceReportFINALMarch25.pdf
Consumer Report July 2013, p. 21

[19] À Aimer. *Getting Sick, Part Four:*
http://foreignparts.typepad.com/foreign_parts/2009/10/à-aimer-getting-sick-part-four.html; *Cost Sharing for Health care: France, Germany, and Switzerland:*
http://www.kff.org/insurance/upload/7852.pdf

[20] *Current Population Survey:* **http://www.census.gov/cps/data/** (the 2012 CPS presents data for 2011)

[21] *RAND Analysis:* http://www.clinical-innovation.com/topics/technology-management/rand-house-bill-could-halve-us-uninsured-2019

[22] *Health Insurance navigator:* http://blogs.webmd.com/health-insurance-navigator/

[23] *Coverage Denied: How the Current Health Insurance System Leaves Millions Behind:* http://www.healthreform.gov/reports/denied_coverage/index.html

[24] *2.5 Million More Young Adults Have Coverage Thanks to Health Law:*
http://www.whitehouse.gov/blog/2011/12/14/25-million-more-young-adults-have-coverage-thanks-health-law

[25] Mary A. Fischer (April/May 2013). *Medical Care You Can Afford:*
http://www.aarp.org/money/budgeting-saving/info-04-2013/medical-care-you-can-afford.html

[26] *States Moving Toward Comprehensive Health care Reform:*
http://www.kff.org/uninsured/kcmu_statehealthreform.cfm